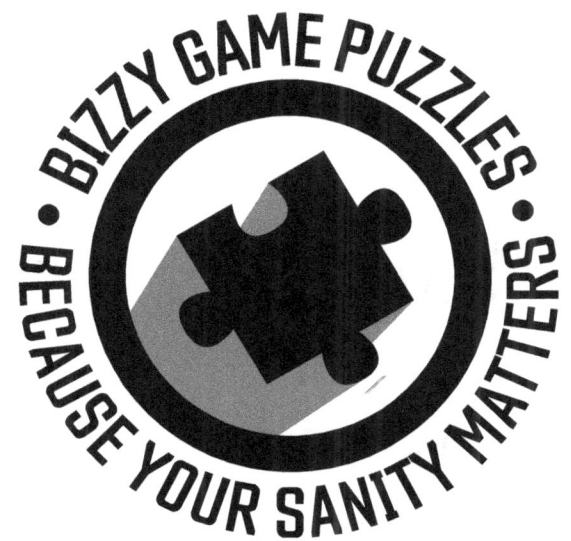

Sudoku Puzzles

200 Unique Sudoku Puzzles

Difficulty Easy

Large Print Puzzles

Large Print Book 8.5 in x 11 in

Answer Key in Back

Page Numbers For Easy Reference

Hours of Entertainment

Sudoku Puzzle Example

						4	7	3
		2						
5			8	1	7			
	4		5			9		
	9		3		1			
				2		1		
	9	2	4					8
1					8		5	
								9

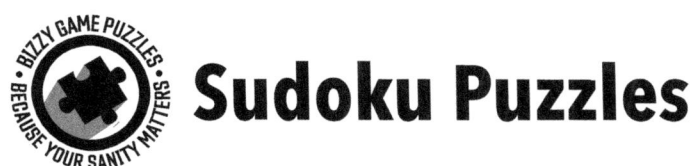
Sudoku Solution Example

8	1	6	9	5	2	4	7	3
9	7	2	6	3	4	5	8	1
5	3	4	8	1	7	2	9	6
2	4	1	5	8	6	9	3	7
6	9	5	3	7	1	8	4	2
3	8	7	4	2	9	1	6	5
7	6	9	2	4	5	3	1	8
1	2	3	7	9	8	6	5	4
4	5	8	1	6	3	7	2	9

Sudoku Instructions

Each Sudoku is comprised of 81 numbers. There are nine horizontal lines and 9 vertical lines, and there are 9 smaller blocks included in each puzzle which are separated by a darker lines.

Rules: Each of the 9 horizontal lines, 9 vertical lines and 9 small blocks include the numbers 1-9, without any numbers being duplicated within the given item.

The challenge is to figure out where the numbers 1-9 should appear in the puzzle, without violating the rules outlined in the paragraph above.

Puzzle# 1

	3		5			2		6
		6	3			1	9	
9	2	7				3		5
7	1	8			2			
	4	2	9			8		
	5		7	1	8			
1		3					6	
2	7		6	3				
	6		2			7	4	3

Solution on Page #101

Puzzle# 2

			8			6		
	7		3	6			4	
8	9		7			1		2
9			6			7	2	1
7	3	2				4	6	
1		4	7					
2	5	7	3		1			
6			9			3	5	
	4				7	2		

Solution on Page #101

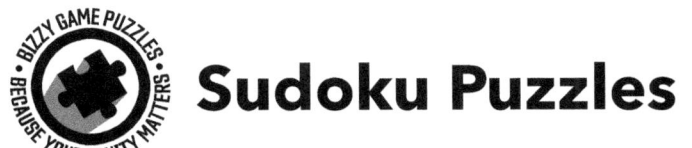

Sudoku Puzzles

Difficulty: Easy

Puzzle# 3

9	7		3		2		1	
	8	3		7	6	2	5	
2			1					
		7			5	6		
	1	8					2	
			6	2			3	8
	4	6						7
	9		5					3
		1	9	6	4	5	8	

Solution on Page #101

Puzzle# 4

4			9					2
	8	6			7		3	
			8	4	3	5		
		1	6			7	4	5
			5			8		3
	5	8	3		4			
				5	6			4
	7	5	4				9	
2	4			8	9	6	5	1

Solution on Page #101

Puzzle# 5

	4		1	6	9			8
8	2				5		6	1
7			4	2				
9	5				4			2
4			2	9			7	
		6	7			8		
		4	9	8				
1		2	5				4	
		3				2	8	7

Solution on Page #101

Puzzle# 6

2		9	8		3	1		
7	8		9					
					2			8
	3		4	8		2		
6	9	8				3		
		5			1			6
5			1		9	7		2
			8	6		4		
	7	3		5	4	9		1

Solution on Page #101

Puzzle# 7

	1	7			2			
		2		5			4	
8		3	6			7	5	2
1				6		2	3	8
3		4			7	9		
	6		5	8	3			7
9			4					
					5	1		
4		8		9			7	6

Solution on Page #102

Puzzle# 8

2			3	1			5	
		7	9		6			3
	4	3			2	9	6	7
4		2	5				7	9
	5	8	2		1			6
	1		7				2	
		1	4					2
9	6				3	7		
		5			9	3		

Solution on Page #102

Sudoku Puzzles

Puzzle# 9

4			5			8	9	
7			4	2		6		3
	5		9		8			
					4		7	6
9			6				2	
	4	5		3	7			9
	6	4	7		2	9		
	2		5					8
	3			6		4	1	

Solution on Page #102

Puzzle# 10

					7			9
3			6	8				
				4	9		3	1
5	1	8			4			6
	4			9	6		1	
			1	2			4	
8		1	4		3		6	
		7		1		3		8
	9	3	5		8			

Solution on Page #102

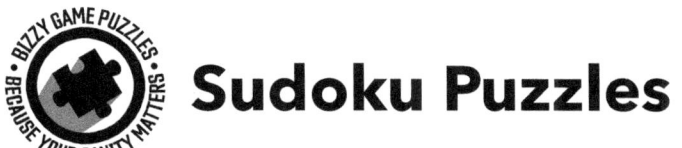

Sudoku Puzzles

Difficulty: Easy

Puzzle# 11

4			6	2	1	8		9
	8						6	
		9		4		3		5
8	5		2				9	
2		1		6	8			
			5			2	8	1
5		3			6		1	
		8	3	5	9	7	4	
	4			7				8

Solution on Page #102

Puzzle# 12

8			4		3		5	
	9			6	2		4	
		6	8	5		1	2	7
2		1				9	3	6
7	3	9	6					4
						2		
			9	8		1		
				6	7	9	2	
	2	4		1		8		3

Solution on Page #102

Puzzle# 13

	3		8	9		5		1
4				7		2		
2		9	6	1				
		1	4		8			9
	8				1	6	7	
3		4			7	8	1	5
	2	3			5		6	
1	4		3	8	6			
	6							7

Solution on Page #103

Puzzle# 14

		9	4	2	6		5	
	8	2			3			
		5		7				
		6				4		
5				4	9			7
	7		3	6				9
1	2		8	9	7		4	
	4	7	6	5	2	1	8	
				3			9	2

Solution on Page #103

Sudoku Puzzles

Puzzle# 15

2		5	7				8	
			2		5			
6		1		4	8		9	2
1	9	2	8					3
	6		5	3		9		
	5				4	1		
	3					2		5
			6	7				4
4	2	8			3		7	

Solution on Page #103

Puzzle# 16

5				9			4	
		9	4		2	5		6
	4			8	6	3		
		2	1				3	9
		5		2			8	
7		6		4				
6			4	8				1
				1		2		8
		8	2	6	5	4		3

Solution on Page #103

Difficulty: Easy

Puzzle# 17

	5		6	8		3		
							2	8
	8	1		.				6
9			1		5	8		
8	1		3	7		5	9	
5		2		9				
1	7		9				4	
			7	4		6	8	
4	6			2	3	1	7	9

Solution on Page #103

Puzzle# 18

					4	7		2
1	4			3		6		
	3	6	.	8				1
		1	5			3		
9			2			4	8	
				4				9
2			3		6			4
	9		8			1	5	
3	5	7	4	1				6

Solution on Page #103

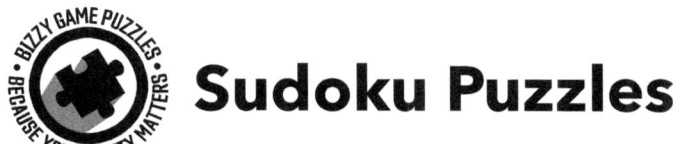

Sudoku Puzzles

Difficulty: Easy

Puzzle# 19

						2	7	6
	1	8						4
	7						3	
9		2	4	8	7	6		
	6		3	9			2	
		2				3		9
6		3		4	9	8		2
				1	3	7	6	5
7					6	9		

Solution on Page #104

Puzzle# 20

			3		8	5		6
9						7		
8		7	4	5	9		1	
			7				3	
	3		2	9	1			
2			6			9		1
3		1	8		2		5	
5	4				7			8
6		8		4		1	2	9

Solution on Page #104

Puzzle# 21

		8	7					9
3		1	5	8	9		6	
					1		4	5
9		7	3			6		
	5					4		7
8			2				5	
6				9	7			4
	7		8			2	1	9
1	8			5	3	2		6

Solution on Page #104

Puzzle# 22

	3						1	6
7	4				2	9		5
	5	8	3			4	2	
	6		5		8			
	2		9	7			5	8
8			4		1	6	9	
4	1				5	2		
							4	9
5			8		3	7	6	1

Solution on Page #104

Puzzle# 23

	8		5	7		4		
				2	4		8	3
4	3	5				6		
3			4		6	7		
		8	7	5	1		4	9
7				3	9		1	
5			3			9		
8				1	5			
	6		8			1		5

Solution on Page #104

Puzzle# 24

2		1			5			
			2				7	
3	4	7		6	1	8		
1			7	2		6	9	
8			5	1	9	3		7
					7	4	3	2
7	2	6	3	4		5	1	
		9		5				6

Solution on Page #104

Sudoku Puzzles

Difficulty: Easy

Puzzle# 25

	5		1			6	7	
2		3			8	9	1	
				9				3
	4	2	9				6	
5		6			7	1	4	
	7		5	6	4		2	8
	2	1		5		4		6
	9	4		2		8		1
			3					2

Solution on Page #105

Puzzle# 26

2			3	6		8		
	9			3			6	
	8			2	4	9		
6	1	9			3			8
			9		7	1		6
4		8					5	
	3			5		6		2
		7			2			
	5	2	3			4	9	1

Solution on Page #105

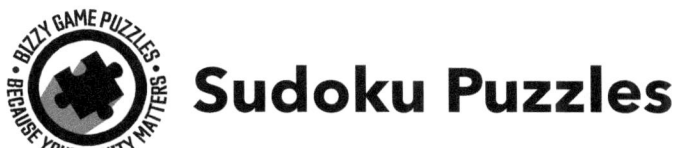

Sudoku Puzzles

Difficulty: Easy

Puzzle# 27

6	7				5	3	2	8
5				3				
3			2	6			9	
		2	6		3	4	8	
	4			2		6	3	
			5	4			7	2
	8		9		2	1	6	
2	6	7			1		5	
1		3	5					7

Solution on Page #105

Puzzle# 28

	6	7		2				9
	4				7			8
2	5	3	9					1
6				7		5		
				4		3		7
4	7		8			9		
3	8	6	5		4	7		2
5	1						6	
					3		4	5

Solution on Page #105

Puzzle# 29

1	4				9		3	
		2		6	7		5	
	6	7	8			1	2	
		9						1
7					1	3	6	
	1			4				
				9		7		2
9			6	1				
8	2	1	3	7	5	9		

Solution on Page #105

Puzzle# 30

		6	9	2		5		
7	1			8		2		
			1		7		3	4
	5	8		4				2
			7		2	9	8	
	3		8	5	9			6
4				7	8	6		1
6		2	4					
		1		9			5	

Solution on Page #105

Puzzle# 31

	5			3	7			2
7	8							
1	2	3	8		4			7
		1	5			2	4	
	6	7	3	4		9	8	
	4		6		9			
	9			2		6	5	8
2	1			6				3
6		5			3			

Solution on Page #106

Puzzle# 32

		3	6	2	4	7		
	7			1		3	4	6
4				5	3	1		
					2		7	
			4	3				
7						4	8	
6	3		2			8	1	
8	9					6	5	2
2	1	4	8					

Solution on Page #106

Puzzle# 33

2	1		3		9			
	3				7	4		1
5			8	1		9	2	3
	7	1		8			3	2
	5		6	3		7		4
		6	7				8	
			1	7				
		9		2			6	
7		3				5		

Solution on Page #106

Puzzle# 34

5	8			9				
	7				8		6	4
			5	7	6	1		9
	1	5		6	9	8		2
					2			1
			4	1		3	9	7
2	6						3	5
3		7		5				
8	5		9			7		

Solution on Page #106

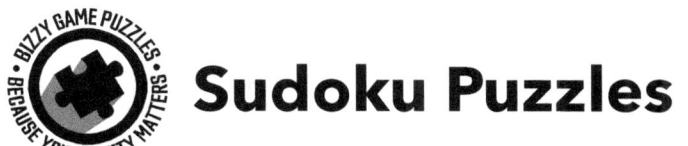
Puzzle# 35

		3				6		
7			6			1		9
9						7		4
	8	9	2			5	7	
4		1		3	7	8		
	5	8	9	6				3
				7	8		5	1
1	4			5	3			7
	9		1	6				

Solution on Page #106

Puzzle# 36

			2		9			
3			8			6	1	7
				7	6		2	3
	1			2	4			
9			3		1		4	2
2		5	7	9		3		
1						4	8	9
4	6	8	9		3			
	9	2						6

Solution on Page #106

Puzzle# 37

2			1		7	5	9	
	7		3	9		4		
		9		4				7
4							7	
	6	3			9	2		
		1			4	8		3
	5	6		3	8	7		9
		7	4		5		3	8
	4		9	7	1		2	

Solution on Page #107

Puzzle# 38

		9	1					
1			8	3			4	6
	6		4					8
6	5	7			2			1
9	3		7	4			5	2
		1				7		
7	9	3		6			1	
		4				8		9
2	8			1		5	3	

Solution on Page #107

Puzzle# 39

6			2		4	5	7	
		7		6			3	
3	4		5			6		
				8		4	9	
	9					1		8
	8				2	7		6
		9	8	1		3	6	7
5	3		9	4				2
		1		2	6			5

Solution on Page #107

Puzzle# 40

9		5	1			2	4	
	2		5				6	1
			6	7	2	5		9
5					8	3		4
				1	5	6		
6	3		9	4		1		5
	1							
		6	8			4	2	
2		8		3		7		

Solution on Page #107

Difficulty: Easy

Puzzle# 41

					4			6
5	7		6	3		9	2	
9			8					4
				8		6		
4			6	9			3	2
	2	8	7				9	
	9	5		8	6			
	1	4	9	7				3
8			1	6	2	7		

Solution on Page #107

Puzzle# 42

	8		4	1		9		
9	6			5			4	
7				6		5		8
		8			3		2	4
		6		2				5
2			6			1	9	3
8	1				5		3	
3	7			1		2		
	2	9	7				4	5

Solution on Page #107

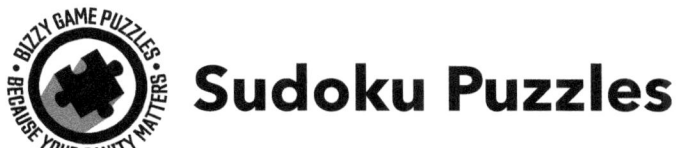

Sudoku Puzzles

Difficulty: Easy

Puzzle# 43

	5				2		7	9
3	1					2		8
	9				3		6	
6		1		4	9	7	2	3
		2	3		7			
	7			6		5	8	
			1	5	6			
8				3	4		5	1
	6			2	8			

Solution on Page #108

Puzzle# 44

3	8		6	2			1	
						5	2	9
		5		1	7	3		8
	5			6				3
	6	4	7			2		
			4		8	1		
7	4	6		3			5	
5			1	4	6	8		2
	1	2	5	7			3	

Solution on Page #108

Puzzle# 45

		3		8	5			
5							4	6
	7	2	4					
	5	7	2	6				
1		6		4			2	3
		4	3	9	7			5
6	2				4	1	3	
8	3			7		5		
			6		3	9	8	2

Solution on Page #108

Puzzle# 46

		3			2			
6		7	3	1	8			5
8					5		1	
		8		6		9		3
4					7	8		1
1	3	5				6	7	
7				5	3			9
9			7	4	6	2		8
	6				1			

Solution on Page #108

Puzzle# 47

2			6		9		7	
			8			2		6
3	6		2	1				
5	4	6		7			1	2
	9		4			6	5	
8				5			9	
1		7			5			4
		8	1	9	2	7		
	2			4	3	5		

Solution on Page #108

Puzzle# 48

5			6	1		2		
			9		3	7	5	
			8	5		1		9
6	1			7	8	5		
	2		5	4			6	
	4		2	6			3	1
1	7					6	9	8
8			1	9		3	7	5
				8				

Solution on Page #108

Puzzle# 49

4	7			9		3		5
1	8	2		5				9
	5	3		1		7		
			8	6			5	
	1		9		3			6
6	2			4		9		7
			4			6	7	3
3	4			8		5	9	
2			7					

Solution on Page #109

Puzzle# 50

	9	1		5			2	
4							5	
2					7	9		3
		9	5	8	1	4	7	
8	4	6			9			
5			3			2		
	3		2			8	6	
7		8	6	3				
9			1		8		4	5

Solution on Page #109

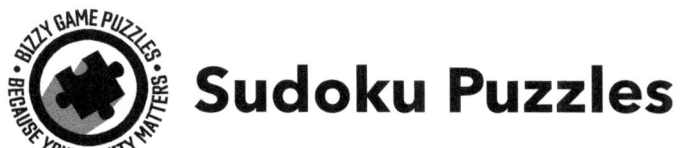

Sudoku Puzzles

Difficulty: Easy

Puzzle# 51

8		7			2		9	4
	9			4	6		8	1
1					8	2	3	
7	4				1		2	9
		6				8		
		8		7	3	5	4	
						7	9	
	8		4		5		7	
2	7	1		8				3

Solution on Page #109

Puzzle# 52

			2	4		9		3
				9	5			
9	7					5	4	1
	9		5	2				6
	1	4	6				9	
	6	5			3			
	9	8				6	7	
	2		7		9			8
5		7	4			3	1	9

Solution on Page #109

Sudoku Puzzles

Puzzle# 53

		9	3					
	5	7			9	2		6
4	2		1				3	
2	1	5			8			
7	3	6				1	8	
9			5	7		6		
		1	7					
			2	1	5		7	4
5		2	4	8				1

Solution on Page #109

Puzzle# 54

	2						8	
		8	4	3	5	7		
			6	8	2			1
	4		1	9	7		5	
3		1			4		6	2
	5			2				
						1	4	3
6				3	5	8	2	
	8				2	9		6

Solution on Page #109

Sudoku Puzzles

Puzzle# 55

	2			7		8	9	
	8					6		5
4		6	9	2		3		
5	7			6	3			1
	1		8	4		7		2
	4	2	7					
	8			5	1			
2	6				7		4	
			4	9	2			

Solution on Page #110

Puzzle# 56

	1	4	2			8		
8	6			7		3		
9	2			3		6		1
			1	5		7		3
1	3		7				8	4
		9			4	1	2	6
	5	2				9	1	
		1		9				
		3	8					5

Solution on Page #110

Puzzle# 57

6			1	5				8
	5			4		1		2
	8					5		9
	2	6					3	4
4			6				8	
	1		4	2	8	7	5	6
1				5	6	4		
5		9				8		
	4				7		2	

Solution on Page #110

Puzzle# 58

	3	9	8					6
6		5		2	7			3
	1		3	5		7		9
				4	2	9		1
		2	7				4	8
		6	1	8	3		7	5
3							9	
5							3	7
	6		4		8	1	5	

Solution on Page #110

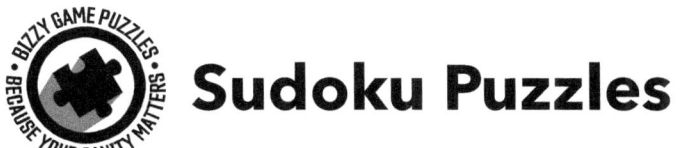

Sudoku Puzzles

Difficulty: Easy

Puzzle# 59

	7		6				8	5
	8			3	4	1	9	
								7
	4			8			6	3
9	1	3	5	6			4	8
	8			3	7			
	9	1		4		5		
4	6	7			1	8		
		5		9				

Solution on Page #110

Puzzle# 60

	1		8			2	3	9
			1	5				4
	2	6	4			5	1	
4						8	9	
	6	7						
9		5	4		3			6
				8		7		
6		8		4		9	5	3
			9	6	7			2

Solution on Page #110

Puzzle# 61

		6					7	9
4	7		8		2		1	
			5	7	6	2		8
8		2		4	5	1		7
3				6				2
			1	2			6	4
					7	4		1
				5				
	1	7	4			3		

Solution on Page #111

Puzzle# 62

2	1		5	6	3	9		
	5		9				6	3
	6				8		1	
3	9		5	7		6		
		5		9		1		2
1	7	6		2			5	
6	3					7		
		9			1	4		
	8	4		3				

Solution on Page #111

Sudoku Puzzles

Difficulty: Easy

Puzzle# 63

			6	8			4	1
		2	1	4	9		3	5
	1	8	2	3				9
3		1			6			2
2	6	7	5			3		
9	8					5		
1	2	3						
						4		8
		6		7	2			

Solution on Page #111

Puzzle# 64

		6	4		8			1
1	3	9						7
		8					6	5
				1		2		
	2	4	7		3			6
5	1			8	2	7		
4	8	1	9			6		3
	6		8		5	4		
9	7				4			

Solution on Page #111

Sudoku Puzzles

Difficulty: Easy

Puzzle# 65

						2	8	
8	7		1			6		9
9		3		4				5
					9	3		6
	1	6		2		8		7
	3					4	5	
	6	4	5	8		9		2
	9	2	6			1		
3			7	2				

Solution on Page #111

Puzzle# 66

3					2		7	5
1	2			7				6
4		7			8	2	9	
9		2	6		3	1		
	6			4				9
	8	3		2				
	1					6		
6			2	8			4	3
			5	9		7	1	2

Solution on Page #111

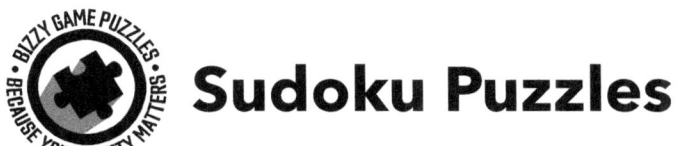

Sudoku Puzzles

Difficulty: Easy

Puzzle# 67

		4	8		6		2	
	5					3		
	2		1		9			
4		1		2		6	8	
		8	9			5	1	
	3			1		4	7	2
					5	9	3	1
3	1	6			4	7		
9	5						6	

Solution on Page #112

Puzzle# 68

					4	5	6	2
		7						
5	2		9		1			
	6			9		1		
		4		8			2	
		8	5			4	7	3
9		5	1	4	3	2		6
4		1		2	8		9	
	8	2	7					4

Solution on Page #112

Sudoku Puzzles

Puzzle# 69

		2	3					
	7		2			9	6	
4			5					3
	7		3		6		5	
		6			7		3	4
		4	8				7	1
7	9			6	3		1	2
			9		2	7		8
2		5		8				6

Solution on Page #112

Puzzle# 70

1		8	6	9				7
	2		5	1				
4		5	3				8	
5	8		4		1	7	3	
2		1				4		
7			9	5			2	8
	5	2		4				9
		4		6			1	
9	1				5	8		

Solution on Page #112

Difficulty: Easy

Puzzle# 71

2		4	7		8			3
8			4	6	3			
				1				
	3				4			9
5			2			4		6
	6	7		3		1		
	4						9	
	5			9			7	4
	7		3	4	5	2	6	1

Solution on Page #112

Puzzle# 72

7	5			4				3
		6			3			
9		8	7	2		5	1	
	6	3		9		1		
2					7	4		5
	7	1		8		6		9
			2					
		4			5	2	7	
8				6	9	3	5	

Solution on Page #112

Puzzle# 73

	3		2	9		8		
	5		6				3	7
4	8	2						1
7		5	2			9	4	3
				1				2
	4	8				5		6
			3				6	8
8	9		4		1	3		
		4			5	7		

Solution on Page #113

Puzzle# 74

4	6		8					9
			6			2		4
7			9	1				
	9	4			2	1	5	
	1	7	3	5				6
3			4			8		7
1	4						3	8
			3	5		4		
5	3	9	4	2			6	

Solution on Page #113

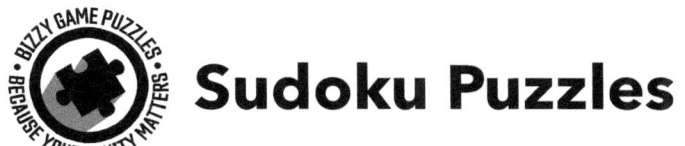

Sudoku Puzzles

Difficulty: Easy

Puzzle# 75

5			4			8		
	9	1						
		4	8	2	9		6	5
9			2				5	
1	6					3		9
	7		1	9			4	
				8	7		3	6
			6	1			2	
6	8		9	4		5	1	7

Solution on Page #113

Puzzle# 76

	6				7			
9			1					5
	2			3	9	1	7	6
2		6	7				5	9
7	1				2	6	8	3
	8	5		9			2	
	9	4		7			1	8
8	5			6				
		1		8	4			

Solution on Page #113

Sudoku Puzzles

Puzzle# 77

			6	4				3
	2		8	5		9		
	9		7	1				5
	4	8	3				1	9
9					1	3		2
	3					7		
		3	1	7	6		9	
8		2		9	5		3	1
6						4		7

Solution on Page #113

Puzzle# 78

5	3			6	8			
2		8	5	9				
		9	2		1	3		
	6			3	4	8		
4			1		2	6	7	
		1	6	7	5			9
	5			1		4	2	6
1								8
	2			5	9			

Solution on Page #113

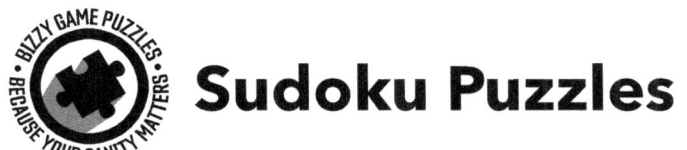

Sudoku Puzzles

Difficulty: Easy

Puzzle# 79

2		7		1	4	8	5	3
	4		3	2				1
		1				2	4	9
	2					9		
6	7				9		1	8
	1	9			8			
	5		7			3		
		2			6			
3	9	4	5	8	1			6

Solution on Page #114

Puzzle# 80

8				5	1	7		
4		6	2	9	7	8		5
1						9		2
9	1		7				5	
2		3	8			1		
	5			3	9			8
5								
	4	9		2			7	
3		7	5		6		4	

Solution on Page #114

Puzzle# 81

		6	5		8			
				1		7		8
8	1				2			
5	9				1	4		7
1				3	4		5	2
	4	7	9		5		3	
3				2			4	5
6			8	4		2		1
			1		7		9	3

Solution on Page #114

Puzzle# 82

	4	2					9	
1		6	7			5	2	
			6		4			
3	1		9			7		
9	7		8			4	6	
6	2						3	
		7		1	9		8	6
8				5		3	4	
		3		7			1	

Solution on Page #114

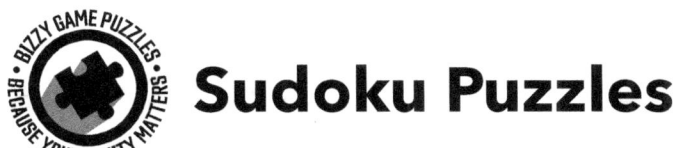

Sudoku Puzzles

Difficulty: Easy

Puzzle# 83

3	1	5		7	2			
	2	8	1	4	6			
6				8		9		
4			6				7	3
1				5			4	
			2	1			6	9
			5			7	3	
	9	6		3				2
7	3	4						5

Solution on Page #114

Puzzle# 84

9			1	4	7		5	
				2	8			
	2					9	8	
3		5					2	9
8	1	9	4				6	
	7	2	5	9	1			4
	3		6				9	
		6	7				4	3
		4		8	3			7

Solution on Page #114

Sudoku Puzzles

Difficulty: Easy

Puzzle# 85

		2	9			7		6
7	4		2			5		9
	9	5			7	4		
					4			3
	6	9			3		8	7
2		8		9	1	6	4	
	5							
9	2						7	1
1		6		7	9	3	5	2

Solution on Page #115

Puzzle# 86

	8	5			9	2		
2		3	5	8				
4	9			3	5			8
			3	5	4			1
1		4	6			8		
	2			1			9	
	1		8			7		9
9		7				4	8	2
				2	7		5	

Solution on Page #115

Difficulty: Easy

Puzzle# 87

	8							9
	2					4		6
	7	9		3	6		1	
	1	7		5			8	
	4		7		9		5	
2			6				9	
1		4	5	6		8		
8	3			9	7	1		5
	6		8	1				3

Solution on Page #115

Puzzle# 88

	9					5		
	5			9		2	4	6
	6		5	3	2	1	9	7
3		9		1			2	
		1	8	4			7	
	8		9					
		2	3	5	9	6		
9	3		4			7	5	
		4			6			8

Solution on Page #115

Puzzle# 89

1		4		6		2		
	2	5	7	4		8		1
5	7						1	
		3	9				4	8
	4	9			8	5		3
3	5	2			7			
4			8	5			2	9
8	9		3	2	6			4

Solution on Page #115

Puzzle# 90

9	6	3		4		2		1
5		2			7	8		4
4	7	8	2				6	
7							4	
	3	9	6	2			5	
		5		1	9	6		
	5			8		4		
		1		7	5		3	6
6							8	

Solution on Page #115

Sudoku Puzzles

Difficulty: Easy

Puzzle# 91

					7		4	6
	9	4		5	3	1		7
8	3		1	6				
	2	8	6					3
		6		1	9	4		8
		1			8			9
		3				6		1
		5				9		
		1		4		6		2

Solution on Page #116

Puzzle# 92

3	9	7		2			4	
	2				6			
	5	4	1	3	9	7		8
2		6			4			
							6	2
4	7	8				1		3
1			9		3	5		6
		3	4				1	
5	6				7		3	

Solution on Page #116

Page #46

Puzzle# 93

3	5						9	
9	2			1			8	4
	4	6	9	2	3	1		
	8							
			8	9		5		
		5	3	4		8		9
5			1					3
4			8			6		7
1			7	9		5	2	

Solution on Page #116

Puzzle# 94

4					3	9		
7			8	5	4		3	2
3		5						
2	3	1	6	4	9	5	7	8
9	5	4						6
	7	8						
	4			9	7		8	
					5		9	
		7	3		6	2		1

Solution on Page #116

Sudoku Puzzles

Difficulty: Easy

Puzzle# 95

2		6						7
	3		4		1	5		
		5	8	7			4	3
	9	1				3	2	
	5	8	7	4				
6	2				3			
5		9	3			8		
1	8		2	5		4		6
	3	2	6			9	1	

Solution on Page #116

Puzzle# 96

5	1					2		
6	3	4	1		2		5	
2				7			4	
3					6	7		
			2	5	9	3	6	8
	8	6		3	1			5
1							8	
	5			1				
7				8		6	3	1

Solution on Page #116

Sudoku Puzzles

Difficulty: Easy

Puzzle# 97

9			4	7	1	3		
3							6	1
		1				8	7	
	3		6	2		5		9
	7				8		1	
	9						8	
7				4		1		
	5	4		1		7		6
8	1		7	6	5	4	9	2

Solution on Page #117

Puzzle# 98

7								
9	8	1				5	6	
3	4				6	9	1	
5			9	4			8	
6	1	3	2		8	4	9	
		4			5	1		
			8		2		4	6
		9		5			3	
					3	2	5	9

Solution on Page #117

Sudoku Puzzles

Puzzle# 99

			4		7			
6	4	3			9			5
	8	2			3		9	
8	1		9	3				7
2		9	5			1	4	
			1	6	4	9		
9	5	8			1		6	
3								9
4		6	7	9	5			

Solution on Page #117

Puzzle# 100

		7					4	
2			4		6		1	8
1		8		5				
	8		7	3			5	
			8		1	6		2
	1				5	8		
8		4					3	
			3	1	4	9		6
6		1	5	9	8			7

Solution on Page #117

Sudoku Puzzles

Difficulty: Easy

Puzzle# 101

	1	5	6					
	4		3	5	2		1	
6	8		1		9	5	2	
		2	8			6		
				1	7	3		2
3			5		6		8	4
5		8		6	3	2		
9		6		8		4	3	

Solution on Page #117

Puzzle# 102

	9	6		1	3			
			6				9	3
1		5	8	9	7	4		6
	1	7						4
2		4	1		8			
				2	6			
		2	9	5	1		4	
6					2			5
5			3			7	1	

Solution on Page #117

Puzzle# 103

		9	5			8		
	4	2	6	8			7	9
7	8			2	9	1		6
9			2					
					7	4	5	
		1		5	6	7		
	7			3	5	9		
5			1				8	
1	3		7		4	2		

Solution on Page #118

Puzzle# 104

	6				3	9		
7				4		2	5	
		5	7	9	1		3	4
5		3						8
	7		9		4		6	
6					8	7	2	9
		6				8		2
	2		1			9	3	
3	5	7				2	1	

Solution on Page #118

Sudoku Puzzles

Difficulty: Easy

Puzzle# 105

7								9
	8	2		6	3			
6		3	5			2	8	
	5	7					1	3
					3			4
8				1		6	2	
2	8		3	9			5	
3			6	1	7			2
9	7		4	2		1	3	

Solution on Page #118

Puzzle# 106

6			2		4			
			1	5			9	
		9			7	1		
	6		7	4			1	
4			1	5	3			
	7		2				5	8
	5		6	2		3	8	9
9		3		1	6			
2	4	6		8			7	

Solution on Page #118

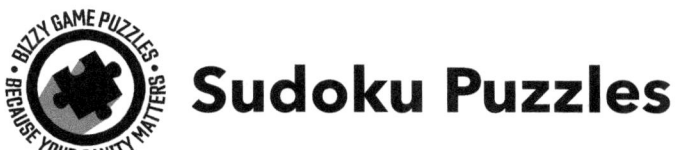

Sudoku Puzzles

Difficulty: Easy

Puzzle# 107

						1	7	
	9		5	1		4		8
2			6			3		
7	4		1					
				9	6			3
6		1	2		7	9	8	4
					1	6	5	
		4	7		5			1
		5			8		4	9

Solution on Page #118

Puzzle# 108

	2	8				7	1	
	7		6	8	2	4	5	
3	4			9		2		
					4			
4		2					8	7
9	3		7	2		6	4	5
			7	1		8		4
	9		8		6	1		
			2		9			

Solution on Page #118

Puzzle# 109

			1	6				4
6		4	3			9	5	
		9	4		2	3		
7				2	3			9
9	5	8						6
3	6				5			7
5		7	8	3	4			2
4					6	1	7	5

Solution on Page #119

Puzzle# 110

6		3	7		4			
7	5			2		4		
	2	4			9		6	
5	9				3	6		
			8		6	9		3
3	6	8	9			2		4
8	3		1	9	2	5		
				3				1
2	1					3		9

Solution on Page #119

Sudoku Puzzles

Difficulty: Easy

Puzzle# 111

		1	7			3		
	2	6		1		8	4	
8	9						2	
			3		2			4
		8			7	6		
	5	2	6		1			
	6		7	2			3	8
2	7	9	8					
	8	4		5			9	7

Solution on Page #119

Puzzle# 112

			7	2	1		8	
		6	3	5				
2					9	7	4	
6		5	1	4		9		3
	8	3						2
1		7		3	2	8		
	1		5	9				8
5		9			3		2	
	4			1			6	

Solution on Page #119

Difficulty: Easy

Puzzle# 113

8	7		6		5			4
	1	9	4	2		3	6	
3			9		8	5	2	
9			1				8	3
		8			9			
			6	3		9	7	2
7		3	8		2		5	1
	9			4			3	6

Solution on Page #119

Puzzle# 114

1			3				7	9
			8	1	4	3		5
	5			7				2
8			9		3	1		
		1			8			
2			1	4		6		
		9			7	2	3	
	2	8			1			6
	1	4				7	5	8

Solution on Page #119

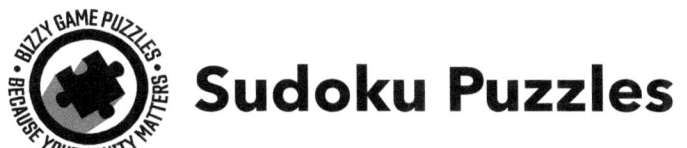

Sudoku Puzzles

Difficulty: Easy

Puzzle# 115

	1	7				3		
				9	6		5	
2								7
	4		8				7	9
6	3	9	2	5		1		4
	8	1	9				3	
1		6	3	4				
8	9	3				4		
		2	5			9	6	3

Solution on Page #120

Puzzle# 116

6			2	9	7			
1	4			8	6	3	9	
3	8	9		5				
		6		2	5			
	1	5			9	4	2	8
2				4		5		
9			5			1		
			4		2	7		
	7	1		9			3	4

Solution on Page #120

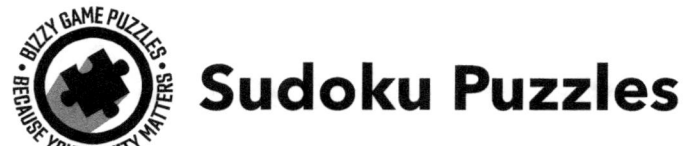

Sudoku Puzzles

Difficulty: Easy

Puzzle# 117

2	4			3	1	9		
		9	8		7		2	3
	3	5		6		7	1	4
		3					4	1
9		1		5			8	
	8				3	6	9	
			6		5			2
4	7				8		5	
1	5		2	7	4			

Solution on Page #120

Puzzle# 118

	1		9	2			6	3
3			8				7	
	6	4	1	3				
7					9	6		8
6	3					5	1	
5	2		4	6	1			
	8	3			2			
		5			4			1
1			7			2	4	5

Solution on Page #120

Page #59

Puzzle# 119

1	7	2	8	4		9		6
5	9	6	1	2				4
3	8	4	9					
				1	9			8
9				3		5		
7		1			6		2	
		7	2	5	4			
6							1	
				9		8	4	

Solution on Page #120

Puzzle# 120

3		6	1		4	5		
			7					
4				5		7		
7					1			
	1	9	4	3	5	8		
		5	9	7	6		1	4
5	6		8			4		9
	8			2		1		7
			5			2	8	6

Solution on Page #120

Sudoku Puzzles

Puzzle# 121

				6	5		7	
		1		7		8		6
		9	4	3	8		1	2
	9	6		4	2		5	
			8			2		
7	2	4			1	3		
	5					9		1
9	6			1			8	
2	1			5	9	6		

Solution on Page #121

Puzzle# 122

	9			2	5		4	
				1				5
5	1	3	8			6	7	2
7	2					5		
		6		5				9
	3		9	6	8			4
9		1	5	7			6	3
4			3				1	7
		7	1		2			

Solution on Page #121

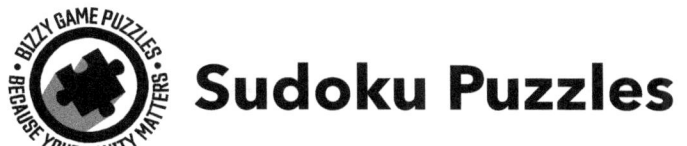

Sudoku Puzzles

Difficulty: Easy

Puzzle# 123

1	4	3	5	8				
6								1
		5	9		1		2	
4	3	8					1	
		9	8	1			7	5
5			2	9				3
3	2	6		4				8
	1	7	3		5	9		
9			6					

Solution on Page #121

Puzzle# 124

6			4		5	3	7	
4	8			2	7	5	6	1
		7	8		3		9	
	4							
5		6			2		8	
			5	3		2	1	
		9		4	1	8		3
						6		7
	2			7	8		4	

Solution on Page #121

Puzzle# 125

		7						
5				3		4		7
		4	7	8	5	9	1	3
4			2			3	5	8
1	3	5	4		8	6		
2				5				
	4		5		3			
	1			4		2	9	5
8			9			1		

Solution on Page #121

Puzzle# 126

	9		6	4	3			2
2			7		9		1	
		7			2	9		6
		9	3	7	8			4
8	3	1	9				6	5
				5	6			8
5	7		2	3			8	9
4		3	8					
				6				

Solution on Page #121

Puzzle# 127

2								
	3	9					8	
				9	2		1	6
	6						5	9
5			9	7	6		2	1
	2	7		4	5			3
	1	8		5	4		9	
7			2		3	6		8
6			7		9	1		

Solution on Page #122

Puzzle# 128

		8			6	3	7	
		3		9	1			
2	9		3		5	4	6	
6					2		9	4
	7	4	9					
	2	5	6			8	1	3
5			2			1		
7						9		
	1		5	6			4	8

Solution on Page #122

Sudoku Puzzles

Difficulty: Easy

Puzzle# 129

4		5	8					
	8		6				5	7
	1				4			
			3				1	8
6			9	2			4	5
	5	2		4		9	6	3
		4		7				
5		8	4		6		7	
3	6		5	8	9		2	4

Solution on Page #122

Puzzle# 130

	4					9	2	
8	6	7	4	2	9	1		5
			6	5		8		4
				8	7			
	3	8	1		6		4	7
6	7	9		3		2	1	
9	1	5						3
7					5		9	
		4		6			5	

Solution on Page #122

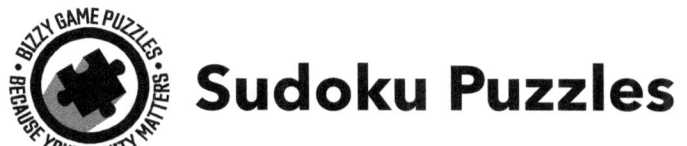
Puzzle# 131

		1						7
	4		9	3	8		5	2
5		9	2		7	4	6	8
3			7	5	6			
9							7	
		8						
7		4	1			5	2	6
2	5	3			9	8	4	1
	8				5			

Solution on Page #122

Puzzle# 132

8			2		5		9	
		6	4		9	1		
		5			1			
		3					4	9
5	6	2				7	8	
9			7	3			1	6
	5	1		2				8
	8			4		6		
3	2	4	6					7

Solution on Page #122

Puzzle# 133

4			6	5			7	
			1			4	2	
			2	9		6		5
5	9		8		7			
	2		5	4		7	9	
	1						6	
	7	9	4		5	8		
6		1		8				
2	5		7	6	1		3	

Solution on Page #123

Puzzle# 134

2				1	5	6	9	
9	7			8		2	5	
					3	7		1
	3		1		9			8
			4				6	
	4			7		3	1	
3	6				7			
4	9	2				8	7	
		8	2		6		3	5

Solution on Page #123

Sudoku Puzzles

Difficulty: Easy

Puzzle# 135

3		9		5	2			
7	5	1		8	6	3		
	4						7	
		5			8	1		
			1	3			5	
1				9		6		4
		4		7				8
		3	2	4	5			7
	9	7		6		2	4	1

Solution on Page #123

Puzzle# 136

	7	3				8		9
	8		6			5	1	
		9	7		4		6	
	6	4			9		8	
				5		7		
3		1	4	7	8	2	9	
1		5		4	7			
			2		1	4		3
	4		8				7	

Solution on Page #123

Sudoku Puzzles

Difficulty: Easy

Puzzle# 137

4		2			5	3	1	
	8				6			4
7				1	9			
8	7	6	1	2	4			
					3			
9	5		7			2		
3	9	1		5		4	8	7
5		7		8		6	9	
	2				7			5

Solution on Page #123

Puzzle# 138

		6	5			9		
3	8			2	7		4	
4		1	9			8		7
9			7	5		2		
	4		3		6	1		
	6		8					5
2		3		1		6	8	
	9	4	2				5	1
	1				9			

Solution on Page #123

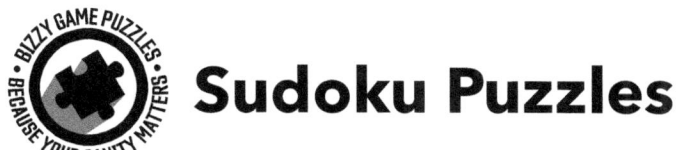

Sudoku Puzzles

Difficulty: Easy

Puzzle# 139

3			2	8	5	4	6	
7		8		1	6			
5	6		7					
1		6						
			3	6	1	5		
		5					7	1
		9			3	8	5	
4	1		8			3		6
	5	3			2			9

Solution on Page #124

Puzzle# 140

4	9						8	2
		2		8	6	5		
		1	4			6	3	7
9						4		
2	6	5	7		8	9		
	4		5	9	3		2	
6		4		7				
	5		9				7	1
7				3				4

Solution on Page #124

Sudoku Puzzles

Difficulty: Easy

Puzzle# 141

	2	1	9			7	6	
8							4	9
3	4			8				
2	6				9	8		
4				7				6
	5		1		4			7
		4		3				1
1	3	2	7			4	8	
6				1	2	9	7	

Solution on Page #124

Puzzle# 142

4		9	3					1
3				9				
	6		4		1	7		
1		7			3		6	
		8			6		4	7
6			9		5	1		8
7		1		8		6		3
9		6	7	3			1	
			6	1		5	7	

Solution on Page #124

Sudoku Puzzles

Difficulty: Easy

Puzzle# 143

7	9			1	5	2	6	
6	1					5	3	
4			6	3	2			
1	6	4		7	3		8	5
	2	7					1	
8			1		6			
		1		6		8	7	2
5			3					
2			8			1		

Solution on Page #124

Puzzle# 144

7	9			3			5	
					7			6
		8	2		9	1		3
6	1					8		
	4	9				6	3	7
	8	5	9	7		2	1	
	3	2	7				4	
			5					
1		4	8			7	6	

Solution on Page #124

Sudoku Puzzles

Difficulty: Easy

Puzzle# 145

2		1		9	3			
8	6	5		7	1		2	
3						1	5	
				3		2	9	
				2		5		8
5	2		9		8	7	4	
	3			6				
1	5	9	3	4				7
	7					4		2

Solution on Page #125

Puzzle# 146

6		4	1			5	2	
7			5	9		4		
	3				8	1		6
	3	6	9	4			1	
2	5							7
			2	3		9		
	4				2		9	1
9								2
1		8				7	3	4

Solution on Page #125

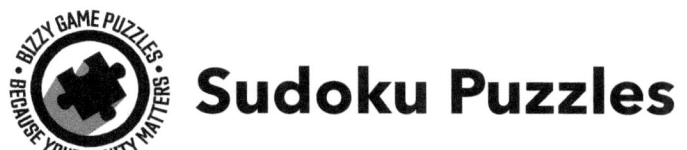

Sudoku Puzzles

Difficulty: Easy

Puzzle# 147

			3	1	8	4	6	
		4	2					9
6		8			9	3		
	4	6				5	8	7
9			8					
8	3				6			1
				3		7	5	
7					4	1		
2	6		1	8	7	9	3	

Solution on Page #125

Puzzle# 148

3		6		8			2	
	9		4	3	2			7
			7	9				
9			5	7		8		1
	1	5			4			9
			9	1		2	6	
	8	4			7			2
6	5		2	4		3		
	2				9			6

Solution on Page #125

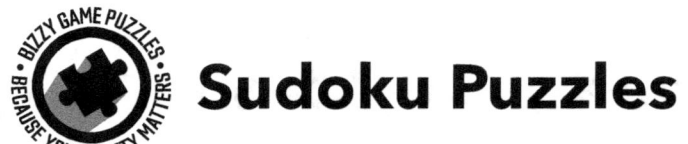

Sudoku Puzzles

Difficulty: Easy

Puzzle# 149

1	8		5		9			
7	4				8	6		
	9				2	8	1	
9	5			2			8	
				7			4	3
8	7		6		4			1
6				4		5	7	8
	1			8		4	3	
		8						

Solution on Page #125

Puzzle# 150

		6		1		9		
4	5		3	8				
				4			8	5
		8	9			6	7	
	9			6	5		3	
		7	4	3		1		9
	6			9		4		
	4	3			2		9	
2		9			4		6	3

Solution on Page #125

Puzzle# 151

		5	8					
		1	5		9	4		2
8	3		7	2		5	1	9
		9						5
4		8		6				
	1	7	2				4	
					7	6	9	
	8	6	1			2	3	7
	7	3	6	9				

Solution on Page #126

Puzzle# 152

		5	6				4	
	9		3		4	5	7	6
			7					1
	8	4		7		6		
		2		4		1	5	
	3		2				9	7
	4	6			7		1	9
8				9	6	3		
	5	9	8		2			4

Solution on Page #126

Puzzle# 153

7			6					2
2	1			4	8	6		
8		5	2				4	
		6				3	9	
1	3	2					8	
		9	7		6	2		5
	4			2	5	1		
			3	1	7	4		
		1			9	5	7	8

Solution on Page #126

Puzzle# 154

			1		9	6		8
			6	2		5	3	
8								2
1	9		4					
6	8			3	1			9
		4			2			6
	7	6	2	8		3		
3	1	5	9	6	7	8	2	4
4	2				3			

Solution on Page #126

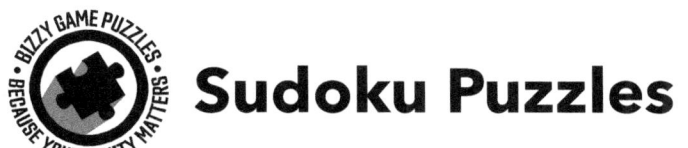

Sudoku Puzzles

Difficulty: Easy

Puzzle# 155

			9	3	1			2
1	2	7			4	3		
				2		5		8
		5		8				3
	8	5		6			2	1
		4	2	1	7	6	8	
5				7				
8						1	2	
4	1		6	8				

Solution on Page #126

Puzzle# 156

7		8	4	1			9	3
6				8	3	2		
4	1		9	6	2	5		
5				9		3		7
	3					4		
		7	3				8	5
						8	3	9
	8		1	2	9			
9			8				4	

Solution on Page #126

Page #78

Sudoku Puzzles

Difficulty: Easy

Puzzle# 157

	7		3			9		4
	3		7			8		
5			9	2		7		1
			5	3			8	
4				7		5	1	
	5						2	
2		7	4	1			9	
6	1	4		9	5			8
	3		7		2			

Solution on Page #127

Puzzle# 158

3		7	6		4			1
	9	1			8			
	5	4				6	7	
		3					4	6
		9	2	6	5	8		
			4			2	9	
7			1	8	6		2	
	3	8		9	2	5		
	6	2		7				

Solution on Page #127

Puzzle# 159

	3			2			8	
	9			3	7			
			9	6		1		3
7	1	2					6	
5	6			8	2	4		
	8		6		3	5	2	
		9	7		5	8	3	
3		8		4				
2			3	9	8			6

Solution on Page #127

Puzzle# 160

		6			9	5	4	
9						7		8
8	4		5	6	1	9	3	
		1	3					
	2		9	1	6			
	9					6	1	
		9	6	2				
	5	4	1	9		2	8	
1			4	7	5	3		

Solution on Page #127

Puzzle# 161

4		3				6	7	8
1			8	7	3		4	
7			9					3
	5	6						1
				2				
	4		1					9
	3	9	2	5		1		
5				6	1			4
2	1		7		8	3	5	

Solution on Page #127

Puzzle# 162

	1		3			9		4
6		8			4		5	3
	9			5				
3		1	4	7		6		5
		4	6			8	7	
7					2			
	3	5			8	4		
	4		9	3		7		
9	2			4	6		3	8

Solution on Page #127

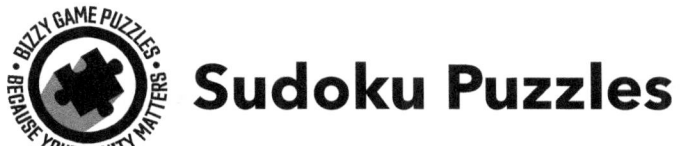

Sudoku Puzzles

Difficulty: Easy

Puzzle# 163

6	2		5	1				
		7	9			5		
1		4			8		2	
7		1			4	3		2
	6					8		5
		5	2				9	7
3	7	8			6			1
			3					
5	4	6		2	1	9	8	

Solution on Page #128

Puzzle# 164

	1	8		6				
9	4	2	7			8	6	
		6				7		
		3	8	1	4			
1		7	6	2			5	
	8			5			3	2
							8	4
		1		8	5	6	9	
	7	5		9			2	1

Solution on Page #128

Puzzle# 165

		7				3	9	4
	4		7	8				1
9		2			4	8		6
4			9	6		2		7
	7	1	4					
6			5	2		1		
1	9	5	6	4				
8				7	2			
7							1	3

Solution on Page #128

Puzzle# 166

	5	2	8			1	9	
7	4				3			6
		1		5				
4				6			8	1
5	8		3	2		4		9
	1	3		8	4			5
					6		3	8
			1			9		
8			4	3		7		

Solution on Page #128

Puzzle# 167

6		7	4	3			8	
3	4	1			6	7		5
		5	7				4	6
2	6							3
	7				2	8	6	
			3				4	5
			6		1	9	3	
			8	2				
7	1		9	5			2	

Solution on Page #128

Puzzle# 168

7			9	4		6		
1	2							5
9			5		6	2	8	
		2		9	5		7	6
6			1		7			
		8			4		2	
	6			5		7		
	4		3		9	5	1	
3		9	2					4

Solution on Page #128

Sudoku Puzzles

Difficulty: Easy

Puzzle# 169

3							6	1
	4		3	8		9	7	
5	7				9			
2	8			3	1	6		
9	6		5	4				2
1				2			5	
7					3		4	
		2	5	4				6
		6	9		1			8

Solution on Page #129

Puzzle# 170

9	4			7				
	2	5		3	4	8	7	
			5		2		1	9
2					7	9		
				2	1	3		
	5	6	4	9				1
7			2	6			5	
			8					
8		9	7	1		2		3

Solution on Page #129

Page #85

Puzzle# 171

4	6	1	8					
			3	9	2	4		6
9			6	1			5	
7	2	5		8			4	
		4	5		1			
6	1		4	3	7			
	4	9				2		
8	7	3				1		
	5			4	3		7	

Solution on Page #129

Puzzle# 172

		1		2	8		3	
8	3		9		6			
		9			4			
			2	4	5	6		
		7		9	1			3
		6		8	3	2	9	
7	1							6
9	2			6	7		1	8
	6		1	5	2			4

Solution on Page #129

Sudoku Puzzles

Difficulty: Easy

Puzzle# 173

	9		3		4	2		
		2	7			6	4	3
4		3					7	1
1		6	2	5				
9	2	4						5
	3		1		6	7		
3		9			5		8	
6						5	2	
	4	5						

Solution on Page #129

Puzzle# 174

	6	9				5		1
	8				6	7		3
	7		5	1		9	6	2
		7		2	1		9	5
	3	1		8	9			7
					5		3	
	2	3				4		6
7			9	3		2	5	
							7	

Solution on Page #129

Puzzle# 175

	7	5			4		3	
	2		3			8		1
	9			2			7	
	3	4	6	7	9	1		
	1		2			5		4
				5	1	7	2	
	3			1	8			7
		7	6	3				9
		6				3		

Solution on Page #130

Puzzle# 176

		3		5	2			
					9		8	
9	7	6			4			
3	4			6				
			8	2			9	4
1		8	4		3		6	7
7				3	5	6	2	1
6						7	3	5
	3	5	7			9		8

Solution on Page #130

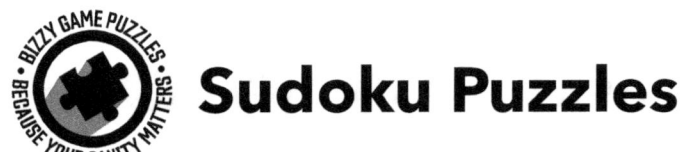

Sudoku Puzzles

Difficulty: Easy

Puzzle# 177

		3	4				7	
	7	8			3			
4	2	6			5	3	1	9
7			2	9		6		5
2	6		1	7				4
9		4			6	7		
3		2	6			8		
		9	8	2				3
	4		3				9	6

Solution on Page #130

Puzzle# 178

8		1	9	7				
4	3		2	6		9	8	
9		6	3	5	8	2		4
			5					
		3			9	7		6
			7		2	8		5
			8				7	9
						3		
2	5		1				4	8

Solution on Page #130

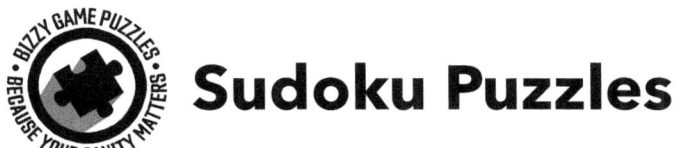
Puzzle# 179

	1	2	5	3		7	4	6
							5	8
	3	4		6	8	2		
		5	3	8	7			2
		3	6	9		1		4
6					1	5		
	6				2			9
2		8	9	7			1	
		7			3			5

Solution on Page #130

Puzzle# 180

			8		2	5		4
1				5				
4	5			3	9	1	6	
				4				
8	9	2	5			4	1	
7		1		9	8	3		
3		6	9			8	4	
		5	3		4			
9					5	7	2	3

Solution on Page #130

Sudoku Puzzles

Puzzle# 181

	5				4		1	
	2	3						
7			8	3		2	5	6
	6	8	3	5		9	2	
		7		8			3	
4						6	8	
3		1	6	7				
5	4			9	8			3
		2		4	3	8		

Solution on Page #131

Puzzle# 182

				9				1
7	8	6			4		2	
			6	8				7
6		4	3					
9	2		8	7	6		4	5
		7			1			6
2	6	3			5		7	4
1	9	8			7			
	7	5		6		1		

Solution on Page #131

Puzzle# 183

	1		3		6	5	4	
	5	3	8		7			
	9	6		4		3		1
	6			8	4	9	7	
8		4		3				
	3	9	2	7				
3				6		8		
	8					7	9	2
9	4				8			

Solution on Page #131

Puzzle# 184

		1				7		
				3				4
8	6		1		7		3	
2		3			8		5	
1					4	6	7	
4	5	6	7	9		1		
	1		4	8			9	7
7		2		6		5		8
3	4	8	5					

Solution on Page #131

Difficulty: Easy

Puzzle# 185

		8		5	6			
1	4			7			2	3
7			3	6		9		
				8	7			1
8	7		6	5				
				1				6
4	8				2	1		9
5		2	7	9		8		4
	6		4	1			7	

Solution on Page #131

Puzzle# 186

	5					1	2	
1		8						
7	3	2			1			8
2		6	1					
	1		6		4		7	2
	8			2	9			3
	6	3	2					1
9			3		7	8		5
	7	1		4		2	3	9

Solution on Page #131

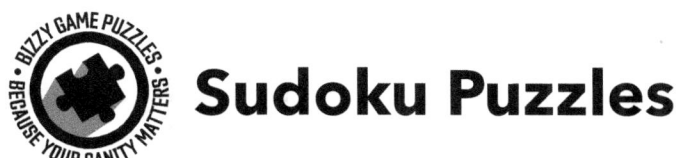

Sudoku Puzzles

Difficulty: Easy

Puzzle# 187

	4	9	7	5	3	2	6	
	3	5		8	6			4
7					1			8
6		2		3	8	7	4	
	7	8		6	2	1	9	
	5			4	7	6		
						8		
							5	6
9	6					3		7

Solution on Page #132

Puzzle# 188

9	8		1		5			
			4				8	5
	3		7	8				
4	9				1	2	5	
	7	8		6	2		4	1
		2	9		7	8		
7				1	8	5		2
6	2				4		9	
				7				4

Solution on Page #132

Page #94

Puzzle# 189

	7			1		9		
2			3	7				
6		9						8
1	9	3	8			7	2	5
4	6	2	5		3		9	1
		7		2			6	
			7	8		4		3
7	1					6		8
					1			

Solution on Page #132

Puzzle# 190

	1	2	7		4	5		
6		7					1	
5	8			2	3			7
9	7	4	2			1	8	3
2	5				1		6	4
			4					
	9					7	4	
		1				2	8	
		6				5	9	3

Solution on Page #132

Difficulty: Easy

Puzzle# 191

	6		8	3	7	4		
		8	4	2	5	1	6	
				6		8	5	
		3						9
	4		6					8
6		9	2			5		
	1			9	6		4	
4	9			8				6
	3	6	5	7		9		

Solution on Page #132

Puzzle# 192

1		3					4	
		8			7		2	
7				5	6	1	8	
	1				4	6		
4		2	5					
8			1	7	3	2		4
			9			3		7
		7	6			5		
	5		7	3	8	4		

Solution on Page #132

Sudoku Puzzles

Difficulty: Easy

Puzzle# 193

2		7					1	
	5	1	7		4	3		9
9				6				
5			2		1			7
1		4			6		3	
7			9	4		2	5	
		9		8	2			5
							9	2
8	1	2		5		6		3

Solution on Page #133

Puzzle# 194

	5		7		4		6	
				1		5		
7	8		2	9				
		2	9				3	7
			8	3			1	
3			4	5		6		
2	7				8			3
9	6	5		2				
8		4		7			2	6

Solution on Page #133

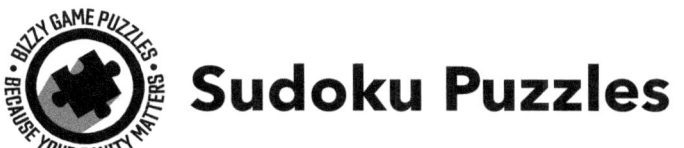

Sudoku Puzzles

Difficulty: Easy

Puzzle# 195

7		1		2				
	5	4						
	8	2			6			4
			5	1	2			9
5					3	4		
1		3	8			7	6	
		7	2		1	5	9	6
	6	5	4	9	7		3	1
2		9	6		5			7

Solution on Page #133

Puzzle# 196

5		3	1		6	4		2
2	4		8	7			9	5
		2			7	6	3	
	7	3	1	9	2			
			5		6			1
8						7	9	
	1							
7			6			5	4	
	9	5	3			1		

Solution on Page #133

Puzzle# 197

1			4	7	5			
7	4				8		6	
9	8		1			7		
4	5	1		2	3	6		8
		3	9		5		4	
	9				1	3		2
			8					
	2	4		1			7	3
3	1		6		4	9		

Solution on Page #133

Puzzle# 198

			1			7		9
		9	8		2			3
3	1	7						
1				2			7	5
9		3				6	2	4
5	4		6					
4	9			3			1	2
2	8			1				7
	3		2	5			6	

Solution on Page #133

Puzzle# 199

4		5	1		2			6
				3				5
	1			6	5			4
	9		6				5	7
1		2		9				3
	4		2	5		1	8	9
			5					8
9	6			1			7	2
5			4	7		6		1

Solution on Page #134

Puzzle# 200

3	4	9					1	2
2	5			4			9	
8	1	6	5			7		
5	6		1				8	
9		8		5		4		
	2	4	8		9	3		6
		2		1		8		3
7						2		
4				8				

Solution on Page #134

Sudoku Puzzle Solutions

Puzzle # 1

4	3	1	5	7	9	2	8	6
5	8	6	3	2	4	1	9	7
9	2	7	1	8	6	3	4	5
7	1	8	4	6	2	5	3	9
6	4	2	9	5	3	8	7	1
3	5	9	7	1	8	6	2	4
1	9	3	8	4	5	7	6	2
2	7	4	6	3	1	9	5	8
8	6	5	2	9	7	4	1	3

Puzzle # 2

4	2	3	1	8	9	6	7	5
5	7	1	2	3	6	9	4	8
8	9	6	4	7	5	1	3	2
9	8	5	6	4	3	7	2	1
7	3	2	5	1	8	4	6	9
1	6	4	7	9	2	5	8	3
2	5	7	3	6	1	8	9	4
6	1	8	9	2	4	3	5	7
3	4	9	8	5	7	2	1	6

Puzzle # 3

9	7	4	3	5	2	8	1	6
1	8	3	4	7	6	2	5	9
2	6	5	1	8	9	3	7	4
3	2	7	8	9	5	6	4	1
6	1	8	7	4	3	9	2	5
4	5	9	6	2	1	7	3	8
5	4	6	2	3	8	1	9	7
8	9	2	5	1	7	4	6	3
7	3	1	9	6	4	5	8	2

Puzzle # 4

4	3	7	9	6	5	1	8	2
5	8	6	1	2	7	4	3	9
1	9	2	8	4	3	5	6	7
3	2	1	6	9	8	7	4	5
9	6	4	5	7	2	8	1	3
7	5	8	3	1	4	9	2	6
8	1	9	2	5	6	3	7	4
6	7	5	4	3	1	2	9	8
2	4	3	7	8	9	6	5	1

Puzzle # 5

3	4	5	1	6	9	7	2	8
8	2	9	3	7	5	4	6	1
7	6	1	4	2	8	3	5	9
9	5	7	8	1	4	6	3	2
4	3	8	2	9	6	1	7	5
2	1	6	7	5	3	8	9	4
6	7	4	9	8	2	5	1	3
1	8	2	5	3	7	9	4	6
5	9	3	6	4	1	2	8	7

Puzzle # 6

2	5	9	8	6	3	1	4	7
7	8	4	9	1	5	6	2	3
3	6	1	4	7	2	5	9	8
1	3	7	6	4	8	2	5	9
6	9	8	5	2	7	3	1	4
4	2	5	3	9	1	8	7	6
5	4	6	1	3	9	7	8	2
9	1	2	7	8	6	4	3	5
8	7	3	2	5	4	9	6	1

Sudoku Puzzle Solutions

Puzzle # 7

5	1	7	3	4	2	6	8	9
6	9	2	7	5	8	3	4	1
8	4	3	6	1	9	7	5	2
1	7	5	9	6	4	2	3	8
3	8	4	1	2	7	9	6	5
2	6	9	5	8	3	4	1	7
9	5	1	4	7	6	8	2	3
7	2	6	8	3	5	1	9	4
4	3	8	2	9	1	5	7	6

Puzzle # 8

2	9	6	3	1	7	8	5	4
5	8	7	9	4	6	2	1	3
1	4	3	8	5	2	9	6	7
4	3	2	5	6	8	1	7	9
7	5	8	2	9	1	4	3	6
6	1	9	7	3	4	5	2	8
3	7	1	4	8	5	6	9	2
9	6	4	1	2	3	7	8	5
8	2	5	6	7	9	3	4	1

Puzzle # 9

4	1	2	3	5	6	8	9	7
7	9	8	4	2	1	6	5	3
3	5	6	9	7	8	2	4	1
2	8	3	1	9	4	5	7	6
9	7	1	6	8	5	3	2	4
6	4	5	2	3	7	1	8	9
8	6	4	7	1	2	9	3	5
1	2	9	5	4	3	7	6	8
5	3	7	8	6	9	4	1	2

Puzzle # 10

1	2	4	3	5	7	6	8	9
3	7	9	6	8	1	4	2	5
6	8	5	2	4	9	7	3	1
5	1	8	7	3	4	2	9	6
7	4	2	8	9	6	5	1	3
9	3	6	1	2	5	8	4	7
8	5	1	4	7	3	9	6	2
4	6	7	9	1	2	3	5	8
2	9	3	5	6	8	1	7	4

Puzzle # 11

4	3	5	6	2	1	8	7	9
7	8	2	9	3	5	1	6	4
6	1	9	8	4	7	3	2	5
8	5	4	2	1	3	6	9	7
2	9	1	7	6	8	4	5	3
3	6	7	5	9	4	2	8	1
5	7	3	4	8	6	9	1	2
1	2	8	3	5	9	7	4	6
9	4	6	1	7	2	5	3	8

Puzzle # 12

8	1	2	4	7	3	6	5	9
5	9	7	1	6	2	3	4	8
3	4	6	8	5	9	1	2	7
2	5	1	7	8	4	9	3	6
7	3	9	6	2	1	5	8	4
4	6	8	9	3	5	2	7	1
6	7	3	2	9	8	4	1	5
1	8	5	3	4	6	7	9	2
9	2	4	5	1	7	8	6	3

Sudoku Puzzle Solutions

Puzzle # 13

7	3	6	8	9	2	5	4	1
4	1	8	5	7	3	2	9	6
2	5	9	6	1	4	7	8	3
6	7	1	4	5	8	3	2	9
5	8	2	9	3	1	6	7	4
3	9	4	2	6	7	8	1	5
9	2	3	7	4	5	1	6	8
1	4	7	3	8	6	9	5	2
8	6	5	1	2	9	4	3	7

Puzzle # 14

7	1	9	4	2	6	3	5	8
4	8	2	5	1	3	9	7	6
3	6	5	9	7	8	2	1	4
2	9	6	7	8	5	4	3	1
5	3	1	2	4	9	8	6	7
8	7	4	3	6	1	5	2	9
1	2	3	8	9	7	6	4	5
9	4	7	6	5	2	1	8	3
6	5	8	1	3	4	7	9	2

Puzzle # 15

2	4	5	7	9	6	3	8	1
9	8	3	2	1	5	7	4	6
6	7	1	3	4	8	5	9	2
1	9	2	8	6	7	4	5	3
8	6	4	5	3	1	9	2	7
3	5	7	9	2	4	1	6	8
7	3	6	4	8	9	2	1	5
5	1	9	6	7	2	8	3	4
4	2	8	1	5	3	6	7	9

Puzzle # 16

5	6	3	7	9	1	8	4	2
8	7	9	4	3	2	5	1	6
2	4	1	5	8	6	3	9	7
4	8	2	1	5	7	6	3	9
1	3	5	6	2	9	7	8	4
7	9	6	3	4	8	1	2	5
6	2	4	8	7	3	9	5	1
3	5	7	9	1	4	2	6	8
9	1	8	2	6	5	4	7	3

Puzzle # 17

2	5	4	6	8	9	3	1	7
6	9	3	5	1	7	4	2	8
7	8	1	2	3	4	9	5	6
9	4	7	1	6	5	8	3	2
8	1	6	3	7	2	5	9	4
5	3	2	4	9	8	7	6	1
1	7	8	9	5	6	2	4	3
3	2	9	7	4	1	6	8	5
4	6	5	8	2	3	1	7	9

Puzzle # 18

5	8	9	1	6	4	7	3	2
1	4	2	7	3	5	6	9	8
7	3	6	9	8	2	5	4	1
4	2	1	5	9	8	3	6	7
9	6	3	2	7	1	4	8	5
8	7	5	6	4	3	2	1	9
2	1	8	3	5	6	9	7	4
6	9	4	8	2	7	1	5	3
3	5	7	4	1	9	8	2	6

Sudoku Puzzle Solutions

Puzzle # 19

5	9	4	1	3	8	2	7	6
3	1	8	6	7	2	5	9	4
2	7	6	9	5	4	1	3	8
9	3	2	4	8	7	6	5	1
8	6	5	3	9	1	4	2	7
1	4	7	2	6	5	3	8	9
6	5	3	7	4	9	8	1	2
4	2	9	8	1	3	7	6	5
7	8	1	5	2	6	9	4	3

Puzzle # 20

1	2	4	3	7	8	5	9	6
9	5	3	1	2	6	7	8	4
8	6	7	4	5	9	2	1	3
4	1	9	7	8	5	6	3	2
7	3	6	2	9	1	8	4	5
2	8	5	6	3	4	9	7	1
3	9	1	8	6	2	4	5	7
5	4	2	9	1	7	3	6	8
6	7	8	5	4	3	1	2	9

Puzzle # 21

5	6	8	7	2	4	3	1	9
3	4	1	5	8	9	7	6	2
7	9	2	6	3	1	8	4	5
9	1	7	3	4	5	6	2	8
2	5	6	9	1	8	4	3	7
8	3	4	2	7	6	9	5	1
6	2	3	1	9	7	5	8	4
4	7	5	8	6	2	1	9	3
1	8	9	4	5	3	2	7	6

Puzzle # 22

2	3	9	7	5	4	8	1	6
7	4	6	1	8	2	9	3	5
1	5	8	3	6	9	4	2	7
9	6	1	5	2	8	3	7	4
3	2	4	9	7	6	1	5	8
8	7	5	4	3	1	6	9	2
4	1	7	6	9	5	2	8	3
6	8	3	2	1	7	5	4	9
5	9	2	8	4	3	7	6	1

Puzzle # 23

2	8	6	5	7	3	4	9	1
1	9	7	6	2	4	5	8	3
4	3	5	1	9	8	6	2	7
3	1	9	4	8	6	7	5	2
6	2	8	7	5	1	3	4	9
7	5	4	2	3	9	8	1	6
5	4	1	3	6	2	9	7	8
8	7	3	9	1	5	2	6	4
9	6	2	8	4	7	1	3	5

Puzzle # 24

2	8	1	4	7	5	9	6	3
6	9	5	2	8	3	1	7	4
3	4	7	9	6	1	8	2	5
1	5	3	7	2	4	6	9	8
8	6	2	5	1	9	3	4	7
9	7	4	8	3	6	2	5	1
5	1	8	6	9	7	4	3	2
7	2	6	3	4	8	5	1	9
4	3	9	1	5	2	7	8	6

Sudoku Puzzle Solutions

Puzzle # 25

9	5	8	1	3	2	6	7	4
2	6	3	4	7	8	9	1	5
4	1	7	6	9	5	2	8	3
8	4	2	9	1	3	5	6	7
5	3	6	2	8	7	1	4	9
1	7	9	5	6	4	3	2	8
7	2	1	8	5	9	4	3	6
3	9	4	7	2	6	8	5	1
6	8	5	3	4	1	7	9	2

Puzzle # 26

2	4	3	6	9	5	8	1	7
5	9	1	7	3	8	2	6	4
7	8	6	1	2	4	9	3	5
6	1	9	5	4	3	7	2	8
3	2	5	9	8	7	1	4	6
4	7	8	2	6	1	3	5	9
1	3	4	8	5	9	6	7	2
9	6	7	4	1	2	5	8	3
8	5	2	3	7	6	4	9	1

Puzzle # 27

6	7	9	4	1	5	3	2	8
5	2	4	8	3	9	7	1	6
3	1	8	2	6	7	5	9	4
7	5	2	6	9	3	4	8	1
9	4	1	7	2	8	6	3	5
8	3	6	1	5	4	9	7	2
4	8	5	9	7	2	1	6	3
2	6	7	3	4	1	8	5	9
1	9	3	5	8	6	2	4	7

Puzzle # 28

8	6	7	4	2	1	5	3	9
9	4	1	3	5	7	6	2	8
2	5	3	9	6	8	4	7	1
6	3	8	1	7	9	2	5	4
1	9	5	2	4	6	3	8	7
4	7	2	8	3	5	9	1	6
3	8	6	5	1	4	7	9	2
5	1	4	7	9	2	8	6	3
7	2	9	6	8	3	1	4	5

Puzzle # 29

1	4	8	2	5	9	6	3	7
3	9	2	1	6	7	4	5	8
5	6	7	8	3	4	1	2	9
4	3	9	5	8	6	2	7	1
7	8	5	9	2	1	3	6	4
2	1	6	7	4	3	8	9	5
6	5	3	4	9	8	7	1	2
9	7	4	6	1	2	5	8	3
8	2	1	3	7	5	9	4	6

Puzzle # 30

8	4	6	9	2	3	5	1	7
7	1	3	5	8	4	2	6	9
5	2	9	1	6	7	8	3	4
9	5	8	6	4	1	3	7	2
1	6	4	7	3	2	9	8	5
2	3	7	8	5	9	1	4	6
4	9	5	3	7	8	6	2	1
6	8	2	4	1	5	7	9	3
3	7	1	2	9	6	4	5	8

Sudoku Puzzle Solutions

Puzzle # 31

4	5	6	1	3	7	8	9	2
7	8	9	2	5	6	3	1	4
1	2	3	8	9	4	5	6	7
9	3	1	5	7	8	2	4	6
5	6	7	3	4	2	9	8	1
8	4	2	6	1	9	7	3	5
3	9	4	7	2	1	6	5	8
2	1	8	9	6	5	4	7	3
6	7	5	4	8	3	1	2	9

Puzzle # 32

1	8	3	6	2	4	7	9	5
5	7	2	9	1	8	3	4	6
4	6	9	7	5	3	1	2	8
3	4	6	1	8	2	5	7	9
9	5	8	4	3	7	2	6	1
7	2	1	5	9	6	4	8	3
6	3	5	2	7	9	8	1	4
8	9	7	3	4	1	6	5	2
2	1	4	8	6	5	9	3	7

Puzzle # 33

2	1	4	3	5	9	8	7	6
9	3	8	2	6	7	4	5	1
5	6	7	8	1	4	9	2	3
4	7	1	9	8	5	6	3	2
8	5	2	6	3	1	7	9	4
3	9	6	7	4	2	1	8	5
6	8	5	1	7	3	2	4	9
1	4	9	5	2	8	3	6	7
7	2	3	4	9	6	5	1	8

Puzzle # 34

5	8	6	1	9	4	2	7	3
1	7	9	2	3	8	5	6	4
4	3	2	5	7	6	1	8	9
7	1	5	3	6	9	8	4	2
9	4	3	7	8	2	6	5	1
6	2	8	4	1	5	3	9	7
2	6	1	8	4	7	9	3	5
3	9	7	6	5	1	4	2	8
8	5	4	9	2	3	7	1	6

Puzzle # 35

8	1	3	7	4	9	6	2	5
7	2	4	6	8	5	1	3	9
9	5	6	3	2	1	7	8	4
3	8	9	2	1	4	5	7	6
4	6	1	5	3	7	8	9	2
2	7	5	8	9	6	4	1	3
6	3	2	4	7	8	9	5	1
1	4	8	9	5	3	2	6	7
5	9	7	1	6	2	3	4	8

Puzzle # 36

6	7	1	2	3	9	8	5	4
3	2	9	8	4	5	6	1	7
8	5	4	1	7	6	9	2	3
7	1	3	6	2	4	5	9	8
9	8	6	3	5	1	7	4	2
2	4	5	7	9	8	3	6	1
1	3	7	5	6	2	4	8	9
4	6	8	9	1	3	2	7	5
5	9	2	4	8	7	1	3	6

Sudoku Puzzle Solutions

Puzzle # 37

2	3	4	1	8	7	5	9	6
8	7	5	3	9	6	4	1	2
6	1	9	5	4	2	3	8	7
4	8	2	6	5	3	9	7	1
7	6	3	8	1	9	2	5	4
5	9	1	7	2	4	8	6	3
1	5	6	2	3	8	7	4	9
9	2	7	4	6	5	1	3	8
3	4	8	9	7	1	6	2	5

Puzzle # 38

8	4	9	1	2	6	3	7	5
1	7	2	8	3	5	9	4	6
3	6	5	4	9	7	1	2	8
6	5	7	3	8	2	4	9	1
9	3	8	7	4	1	6	5	2
4	2	1	6	5	9	7	8	3
7	9	3	5	6	8	2	1	4
5	1	4	2	7	3	8	6	9
2	8	6	9	1	4	5	3	7

Puzzle # 39

6	1	8	2	3	4	5	7	9
9	5	7	1	6	8	2	3	4
3	4	2	5	7	9	6	8	1
2	6	5	7	8	1	4	9	3
7	9	4	6	5	3	1	2	8
1	8	3	4	9	2	7	5	6
4	2	9	8	1	5	3	6	7
5	3	6	9	4	7	8	1	2
8	7	1	3	2	6	9	4	5

Puzzle # 40

9	6	5	1	8	3	2	4	7
3	2	7	5	9	4	8	6	1
1	8	4	6	7	2	5	3	9
5	7	1	2	6	8	3	9	4
8	4	9	3	1	5	6	7	2
6	3	2	9	4	7	1	8	5
4	1	3	7	2	6	9	5	8
7	9	6	8	5	1	4	2	3
2	5	8	4	3	9	7	1	6

Puzzle # 41

3	8	2	9	5	4	7	1	6
5	7	4	6	3	1	9	2	8
9	1	6	8	7	2	3	5	4
1	9	3	2	8	5	4	6	7
4	5	7	1	6	9	8	3	2
6	2	8	7	4	3	1	9	5
7	3	9	5	2	8	6	4	1
2	6	1	4	9	7	5	8	3
8	4	5	3	1	6	2	7	9

Puzzle # 42

5	8	2	3	4	1	9	6	7
9	6	1	8	5	7	3	4	2
7	4	3	9	6	2	5	1	8
1	9	8	5	7	3	6	2	4
4	3	6	1	2	9	8	7	5
2	5	7	6	8	4	1	9	3
8	1	4	2	9	5	7	3	6
3	7	5	4	1	6	2	8	9
6	2	9	7	3	8	4	5	1

Sudoku Puzzle Solutions

Puzzle # 43

4	5	6	8	1	2	3	7	9
3	1	7	6	9	5	2	4	8
2	9	8	4	7	3	1	6	5
6	8	1	5	4	9	7	2	3
5	4	2	3	8	7	9	1	6
9	7	3	2	6	1	5	8	4
7	3	4	1	5	6	8	9	2
8	2	9	7	3	4	6	5	1
1	6	5	9	2	8	4	3	7

Puzzle # 44

3	8	9	6	2	5	4	1	7
6	7	1	3	8	4	5	2	9
4	2	5	9	1	7	3	6	8
9	5	8	2	6	1	7	4	3
1	6	4	7	9	3	2	8	5
2	3	7	4	5	8	1	9	6
7	4	6	8	3	2	9	5	1
5	9	3	1	4	6	8	7	2
8	1	2	5	7	9	6	3	4

Puzzle # 45

4	6	3	1	8	5	2	7	9
5	1	8	7	2	9	3	4	6
9	7	2	4	3	6	8	5	1
3	5	7	2	6	1	4	9	8
1	9	6	5	4	8	7	2	3
2	8	4	3	9	7	6	1	5
6	2	9	8	5	4	1	3	7
8	3	1	9	7	2	5	6	4
7	4	5	6	1	3	9	8	2

Puzzle # 46

5	1	3	4	9	2	7	8	6
6	2	7	3	1	8	4	9	5
8	4	9	6	7	5	3	1	2
2	7	8	1	6	4	9	5	3
4	9	6	5	3	7	8	2	1
1	3	5	8	2	9	6	7	4
7	8	4	2	5	3	1	6	9
9	5	1	7	4	6	2	3	8
3	6	2	9	8	1	5	4	7

Puzzle # 47

2	8	4	6	3	9	1	7	5
9	7	1	5	8	4	2	3	6
3	6	5	2	1	7	8	4	9
5	4	6	9	7	8	3	1	2
7	9	3	4	2	1	6	5	8
8	1	2	3	5	6	4	9	7
1	3	7	8	6	5	9	2	4
4	5	8	1	9	2	7	6	3
6	2	9	7	4	3	5	8	1

Puzzle # 48

5	9	7	6	1	4	2	8	3
4	8	1	9	2	3	7	5	6
2	3	6	8	5	7	1	4	9
6	1	9	3	7	8	5	2	4
3	2	8	5	4	1	9	6	7
7	4	5	2	6	9	8	3	1
1	7	2	4	3	5	6	9	8
8	6	4	1	9	2	3	7	5
9	5	3	7	8	6	4	1	2

Sudoku Puzzle Solutions

Puzzle # 49

4	7	6	2	9	8	3	1	5
1	8	2	3	5	7	4	6	9
9	5	3	6	1	4	7	2	8
7	3	9	8	6	2	1	5	4
5	1	4	9	7	3	2	8	6
6	2	8	5	4	1	9	3	7
8	9	1	4	2	5	6	7	3
3	4	7	1	8	6	5	9	2
2	6	5	7	3	9	8	4	1

Puzzle # 50

6	9	1	8	5	3	7	2	4
4	7	3	9	1	2	6	5	8
2	8	5	4	6	7	9	1	3
3	2	9	5	8	1	4	7	6
8	4	6	7	2	9	5	3	1
5	1	7	3	4	6	2	8	9
1	3	4	2	9	5	8	6	7
7	5	8	6	3	4	1	9	2
9	6	2	1	7	8	3	4	5

Puzzle # 51

8	3	7	5	1	2	6	9	4
5	9	2	3	4	6	7	8	1
1	6	4	7	9	8	2	3	5
7	4	5	8	6	1	3	2	9
3	2	6	9	5	4	8	1	7
9	1	8	2	7	3	5	4	6
4	5	3	1	2	7	9	6	8
6	8	9	4	3	5	1	7	2
2	7	1	6	8	9	4	5	3

Puzzle # 52

8	5	1	2	4	7	9	6	3
6	4	3	1	9	5	8	2	7
9	7	2	3	8	6	5	4	1
7	9	8	5	2	4	1	3	6
3	1	4	6	7	8	2	9	5
2	6	5	9	1	3	7	8	4
4	3	9	8	5	1	6	7	2
1	2	6	7	3	9	4	5	8
5	8	7	4	6	2	3	1	9

Puzzle # 53

1	6	9	3	5	2	7	4	8
3	5	7	8	4	9	2	1	6
4	2	8	1	6	7	5	3	9
2	1	5	6	3	8	4	9	7
7	3	6	9	2	4	1	8	5
9	8	4	5	7	1	6	2	3
8	4	1	7	9	6	3	5	2
6	9	3	2	1	5	8	7	4
5	7	2	4	8	3	9	6	1

Puzzle # 54

4	2	5	7	1	9	6	8	3
1	6	8	2	4	3	5	7	9
7	3	9	5	6	8	2	4	1
2	4	6	1	9	7	3	5	8
3	9	1	8	5	4	7	6	2
8	5	7	3	2	6	1	9	4
9	7	2	6	8	1	4	3	5
6	1	4	9	3	5	8	2	7
5	8	3	4	7	2	9	1	6

Sudoku Puzzle Solutions

Puzzle # 55

3	2	1	5	7	6	8	9	4
7	9	8	1	3	4	6	2	5
4	5	6	9	2	8	3	1	7
5	7	9	2	6	3	4	8	1
6	1	3	8	4	9	7	5	2
8	4	2	7	1	5	9	3	6
9	8	4	6	5	1	2	7	3
2	6	5	3	8	7	1	4	9
1	3	7	4	9	2	5	6	8

Puzzle # 56

3	1	4	2	6	5	8	7	9
8	6	5	9	7	1	3	4	2
9	2	7	4	3	8	6	5	1
2	4	8	1	5	6	7	9	3
1	3	6	7	2	9	5	8	4
5	7	9	3	8	4	1	2	6
7	5	2	6	4	3	9	1	8
6	8	1	5	9	2	4	3	7
4	9	3	8	1	7	2	6	5

Puzzle # 57

6	9	4	2	1	5	3	7	8
7	3	5	9	8	4	1	6	2
2	8	1	7	6	3	5	4	9
8	2	6	5	7	1	9	3	4
4	5	7	6	3	9	2	8	1
9	1	3	4	2	8	7	5	6
1	7	2	8	5	6	4	9	3
5	6	9	3	4	2	8	1	7
3	4	8	1	9	7	6	2	5

Puzzle # 58

7	3	9	8	1	4	5	2	6
6	8	5	9	2	7	4	1	3
2	1	4	3	5	6	7	8	9
8	7	3	5	4	2	9	6	1
1	5	2	7	6	9	3	4	8
4	9	6	1	8	3	2	7	5
3	2	1	6	7	5	8	9	4
5	4	8	2	9	1	6	3	7
9	6	7	4	3	8	1	5	2

Puzzle # 59

3	7	9	6	1	2	4	8	5
5	2	8	7	3	4	1	9	6
1	4	6	9	8	5	3	2	7
7	5	4	1	2	8	9	6	3
9	1	3	5	6	7	2	4	8
6	8	2	4	9	3	7	5	1
8	9	1	3	4	6	5	7	2
4	6	7	2	5	1	8	3	9
2	3	5	8	7	9	6	1	4

Puzzle # 60

5	1	4	7	8	6	2	3	9
8	9	3	2	1	5	7	6	4
7	2	6	3	4	9	5	1	8
4	3	2	6	5	1	8	9	7
1	6	7	8	9	2	3	4	5
9	8	5	4	7	3	1	2	6
2	4	9	5	3	8	6	7	1
6	7	8	1	2	4	9	5	3
3	5	1	9	6	7	4	8	2

Sudoku Puzzle Solutions

Puzzle # 61

2	8	6	3	1	4	5	7	9
4	7	5	8	9	2	6	1	3
1	9	3	5	7	6	2	4	8
8	6	2	9	4	5	1	3	7
3	4	1	7	6	8	9	5	2
7	5	9	1	2	3	8	6	4
5	2	8	6	3	7	4	9	1
9	3	4	2	5	1	7	8	6
6	1	7	4	8	9	3	2	5

Puzzle # 62

2	1	8	5	6	3	9	4	7
4	5	7	9	1	2	8	6	3
9	6	3	4	7	8	2	1	5
3	9	2	1	5	7	6	8	4
8	4	5	3	9	6	1	7	2
1	7	6	8	2	4	3	5	9
6	3	1	2	4	5	7	9	8
5	2	9	7	8	1	4	3	6
7	8	4	6	3	9	5	2	1

Puzzle # 63

5	3	9	6	8	7	2	4	1
6	7	2	1	4	9	8	3	5
4	1	8	2	3	5	6	7	9
3	5	1	4	9	6	7	8	2
2	6	7	5	1	8	3	9	4
9	8	4	7	2	3	5	1	6
1	2	3	8	5	4	9	6	7
7	9	5	3	6	1	4	2	8
8	4	6	9	7	2	1	5	3

Puzzle # 64

2	5	6	4	7	8	9	3	1
1	3	9	2	5	6	8	4	7
7	4	8	1	3	9	2	6	5
6	9	7	5	4	1	3	2	8
8	2	4	7	9	3	5	1	6
5	1	3	6	8	2	7	9	4
4	8	1	9	2	7	6	5	3
3	6	2	8	1	5	4	7	9
9	7	5	3	6	4	1	8	2

Puzzle # 65

6	4	1	9	5	7	2	8	3
8	7	5	1	3	2	6	4	9
9	2	3	8	4	6	7	1	5
7	5	8	4	1	9	3	2	6
4	1	6	3	2	5	8	9	7
2	3	9	7	6	8	4	5	1
1	6	4	5	8	3	9	7	2
5	9	2	6	7	4	1	3	8
3	8	7	2	9	1	5	6	4

Puzzle # 66

3	9	6	4	1	2	8	7	5
1	2	8	9	7	5	4	3	6
4	5	7	3	6	8	2	9	1
9	4	2	6	5	3	1	8	7
5	6	1	8	4	7	3	2	9
7	8	3	1	2	9	5	6	4
2	1	9	7	3	4	6	5	8
6	7	5	2	8	1	9	4	3
8	3	4	5	9	6	7	1	2

Sudoku Puzzle Solutions

Puzzle # 67

7	9	4	8	3	6	1	2	5
1	8	5	4	7	2	3	9	6
6	2	3	1	5	9	8	4	7
4	7	1	5	2	3	6	8	9
2	6	8	9	4	7	5	1	3
5	3	9	6	1	8	4	7	2
8	4	2	7	6	5	9	3	1
3	1	6	2	9	4	7	5	8
9	5	7	3	8	1	2	6	4

Puzzle # 68

3	1	9	8	7	4	5	6	2
8	4	7	2	6	5	9	3	1
5	2	6	9	3	1	8	4	7
7	6	3	4	9	2	1	5	8
1	5	4	3	8	7	6	2	9
2	9	8	5	1	6	4	7	3
9	7	5	1	4	3	2	8	6
4	3	1	6	2	8	7	9	5
6	8	2	7	5	9	3	1	4

Puzzle # 69

1	5	2	6	3	9	4	8	7
3	8	7	2	1	4	9	6	5
4	6	9	5	7	8	1	2	3
8	7	1	3	4	6	2	5	9
5	2	6	1	9	7	8	3	4
9	3	4	8	2	5	6	7	1
7	9	8	4	6	3	5	1	2
6	1	3	9	5	2	7	4	8
2	4	5	7	8	1	3	9	6

Puzzle # 70

1	3	8	6	9	4	2	5	7
6	2	7	5	1	8	9	4	3
4	9	5	3	7	2	6	8	1
5	8	9	4	2	1	7	3	6
2	6	1	7	8	3	4	9	5
7	4	3	9	5	6	1	2	8
8	5	2	1	4	7	3	6	9
3	7	4	8	6	9	5	1	2
9	1	6	2	3	5	8	7	4

Puzzle # 71

2	9	4	7	5	8	6	1	3
8	1	5	4	6	3	9	2	7
7	3	6	9	1	2	5	4	8
1	2	3	6	8	4	7	5	9
5	8	9	2	7	1	4	3	6
4	6	7	5	3	9	1	8	2
6	4	1	8	2	7	3	9	5
3	5	2	1	9	6	8	7	4
9	7	8	3	4	5	2	6	1

Puzzle # 72

7	5	2	9	4	1	8	6	3
1	4	6	8	5	3	7	9	2
9	3	8	7	2	6	5	1	4
4	6	3	5	9	2	1	8	7
2	8	9	6	1	7	4	3	5
5	7	1	3	8	4	6	2	9
3	1	5	2	7	8	9	4	6
6	9	4	1	3	5	2	7	8
8	2	7	4	6	9	3	5	1

Sudoku Puzzle Solutions

Puzzle # 73

6	3	7	1	2	9	8	5	4
1	5	9	6	4	8	2	3	7
4	8	2	7	5	3	6	9	1
7	1	5	2	8	6	9	4	3
9	6	3	5	1	4	7	8	2
2	4	8	9	3	7	5	1	6
5	7	1	3	9	2	4	6	8
8	9	6	4	7	1	3	2	5
3	2	4	8	6	5	1	7	9

Puzzle # 74

4	6	5	2	8	7	3	1	9
9	8	1	5	6	3	2	7	4
7	2	3	9	1	4	6	8	5
8	9	4	6	7	2	1	5	3
2	1	7	8	3	5	9	4	6
3	5	6	1	4	9	8	2	7
1	4	2	7	9	6	5	3	8
6	7	8	3	5	1	4	9	2
5	3	9	4	2	8	7	6	1

Puzzle # 75

5	2	6	4	7	1	8	9	3
8	9	1	3	6	5	2	7	4
7	3	4	8	2	9	1	6	5
9	4	8	2	3	6	7	5	1
1	6	2	7	5	4	3	8	9
3	7	5	1	9	8	6	4	2
2	1	9	5	8	7	4	3	6
4	5	7	6	1	3	9	2	8
6	8	3	9	4	2	5	1	7

Puzzle # 76

1	6	3	8	5	7	2	9	4
9	4	7	1	2	6	8	3	5
5	2	8	4	3	9	1	7	6
2	3	6	7	1	8	4	5	9
7	1	9	5	4	2	6	8	3
4	8	5	6	9	3	7	2	1
6	9	4	2	7	5	3	1	8
8	5	2	3	6	1	9	4	7
3	7	1	9	8	4	5	6	2

Puzzle # 77

7	8	5	6	4	9	1	2	3
1	2	6	8	5	3	9	7	4
3	9	4	7	1	2	8	6	5
2	4	8	3	6	7	5	1	9
9	6	7	5	8	1	3	4	2
5	3	1	9	2	4	7	8	6
4	5	3	1	7	6	2	9	8
8	7	2	4	9	5	6	3	1
6	1	9	2	3	8	4	5	7

Puzzle # 78

5	3	4	7	6	8	9	1	2
2	1	8	5	9	3	7	6	4
6	7	9	2	4	1	3	8	5
7	6	2	9	3	4	8	5	1
4	9	5	1	8	2	6	7	3
3	8	1	6	7	5	2	4	9
9	5	3	8	1	7	4	2	6
1	4	7	3	2	6	5	9	8
8	2	6	4	5	9	1	3	7

Sudoku Puzzle Solutions

Puzzle # 79

2	6	7	9	1	4	8	5	3
9	4	8	3	2	5	6	7	1
5	3	1	8	6	7	2	4	9
8	2	5	1	4	3	9	6	7
6	7	3	2	5	9	4	1	8
4	1	9	6	7	8	5	3	2
1	5	6	7	9	2	3	8	4
7	8	2	4	3	6	1	9	5
3	9	4	5	8	1	7	2	6

Puzzle # 80

8	9	2	6	5	1	7	3	4
4	3	6	2	9	7	8	1	5
1	7	5	4	8	3	9	6	2
9	1	8	7	6	2	4	5	3
2	6	3	8	4	5	1	9	7
7	5	4	1	3	9	6	2	8
5	2	1	9	7	4	3	8	6
6	4	9	3	2	8	5	7	1
3	8	7	5	1	6	2	4	9

Puzzle # 81

7	2	6	5	9	8	3	1	4
9	3	5	4	1	6	7	2	8
8	1	4	3	7	2	5	6	9
5	9	3	2	6	1	4	8	7
1	6	8	7	3	4	9	5	2
2	4	7	9	8	5	1	3	6
3	7	1	6	2	9	8	4	5
6	5	9	8	4	3	2	7	1
4	8	2	1	5	7	6	9	3

Puzzle # 82

7	4	2	1	8	5	6	9	3
1	8	6	7	9	3	5	2	4
5	3	9	6	2	4	8	7	1
3	1	4	9	6	2	7	5	8
9	7	5	8	3	1	4	6	2
6	2	8	5	4	7	1	3	9
4	5	7	3	1	9	2	8	6
8	9	1	2	5	6	3	4	7
2	6	3	4	7	8	9	1	5

Puzzle # 83

3	1	5	9	7	2	4	8	6
9	2	8	1	4	6	3	5	7
6	4	7	3	8	5	9	2	1
4	5	2	6	9	8	1	7	3
1	6	9	7	5	3	2	4	8
8	7	3	2	1	4	5	6	9
2	8	1	5	6	9	7	3	4
5	9	6	4	3	7	8	1	2
7	3	4	8	2	1	6	9	5

Puzzle # 84

9	6	8	1	4	7	3	5	2
1	5	3	9	2	8	4	7	6
4	2	7	3	6	5	9	8	1
3	4	5	8	7	6	1	2	9
8	1	9	4	3	2	7	6	5
6	7	2	5	9	1	8	3	4
7	3	1	6	5	4	2	9	8
2	8	6	7	1	9	5	4	3
5	9	4	2	8	3	6	1	7

Sudoku Puzzle Solutions

Puzzle # 85

8	1	2	9	4	5	7	3	6
7	4	3	2	6	8	5	1	9
6	9	5	1	3	7	4	2	8
5	7	1	6	8	4	2	9	3
4	6	9	5	2	3	1	8	7
2	3	8	7	9	1	6	4	5
3	5	7	8	1	2	9	6	4
9	2	4	3	5	6	8	7	1
1	8	6	4	7	9	3	5	2

Puzzle # 86

7	8	5	4	6	9	2	1	3
2	6	3	5	8	1	9	4	7
4	9	1	2	7	3	5	6	8
8	7	9	3	5	4	6	2	1
1	3	4	6	9	2	8	7	5
5	2	6	7	1	8	3	9	4
6	1	2	8	4	5	7	3	9
9	5	7	1	3	6	4	8	2
3	4	8	9	2	7	1	5	6

Puzzle # 87

3	8	6	1	4	5	2	7	9
5	2	1	9	7	8	4	3	6
4	7	9	2	3	6	5	1	8
9	1	7	3	5	4	6	8	2
6	4	8	7	2	9	3	5	1
2	5	3	6	8	1	7	9	4
1	9	4	5	6	3	8	2	7
8	3	2	4	9	7	1	6	5
7	6	5	8	1	2	9	4	3

Puzzle # 88

2	9	7	1	6	4	5	8	3
1	5	3	7	9	8	2	4	6
4	6	8	5	3	2	1	9	7
3	4	9	6	1	7	8	2	5
6	2	1	8	4	5	3	7	9
7	8	5	9	2	3	4	6	1
8	7	2	3	5	9	6	1	4
9	3	6	4	8	1	7	5	2
5	1	4	2	7	6	9	3	8

Puzzle # 89

1	8	4	5	6	9	2	3	7
7	3	6	1	8	2	4	9	5
9	2	5	7	4	3	8	6	1
5	7	8	6	3	4	9	1	2
2	1	3	9	7	5	6	4	8
6	4	9	2	1	8	5	7	3
3	5	2	4	9	7	1	8	6
4	6	7	8	5	1	3	2	9
8	9	1	3	2	6	7	5	4

Puzzle # 90

9	6	3	5	4	8	2	7	1
5	1	2	3	6	7	8	9	4
4	7	8	2	9	1	3	6	5
7	2	6	8	5	3	1	4	9
1	3	9	6	2	4	7	5	8
8	4	5	7	1	9	6	2	3
3	5	7	9	8	6	4	1	2
2	8	1	4	7	5	9	3	6
6	9	4	1	3	2	5	8	7

Sudoku Puzzle Solutions

Puzzle # 91

1	5	2	9	8	7	3	4	6
6	9	4	2	5	3	1	8	7
8	3	7	1	6	4	2	9	5
9	2	8	6	4	5	7	1	3
5	7	6	3	1	9	4	2	8
3	4	1	7	2	8	5	6	9
4	8	3	5	9	2	6	7	1
2	6	5	8	7	1	9	3	4
7	1	9	4	3	6	8	5	2

Puzzle # 92

3	9	7	5	2	8	6	4	1
8	2	1	7	4	6	3	9	5
6	5	4	1	3	9	7	2	8
2	1	6	3	5	4	9	8	7
9	3	5	8	7	1	4	6	2
4	7	8	6	9	2	1	5	3
1	4	2	9	8	3	5	7	6
7	8	3	4	6	5	2	1	9
5	6	9	2	1	7	8	3	4

Puzzle # 93

3	5	1	4	7	8	2	9	6
9	2	7	5	1	6	3	8	4
8	4	6	9	2	3	1	7	5
7	8	9	6	5	1	4	3	2
6	3	4	2	8	9	7	5	1
2	1	5	3	4	7	8	6	9
5	7	8	1	6	2	9	4	3
4	9	2	8	3	5	6	1	7
1	6	3	7	9	4	5	2	8

Puzzle # 94

4	8	2	1	6	3	9	5	7
7	6	9	8	5	4	1	3	2
3	1	5	9	7	2	8	6	4
2	3	1	6	4	9	5	7	8
9	5	4	7	2	8	3	1	6
6	7	8	5	3	1	4	2	9
1	4	3	2	9	7	6	8	5
8	2	6	4	1	5	7	9	3
5	9	7	3	8	6	2	4	1

Puzzle # 95

2	4	6	9	3	5	1	8	7
8	7	3	4	2	1	5	6	9
9	1	5	8	7	6	2	4	3
7	9	1	5	6	8	3	2	4
3	5	8	7	4	2	6	9	1
6	2	4	1	9	3	7	5	8
5	6	9	3	1	4	8	7	2
1	8	7	2	5	9	4	3	6
4	3	2	6	8	7	9	1	5

Puzzle # 96

5	1	7	4	6	8	2	9	3
6	3	4	1	9	2	8	5	7
2	9	8	5	7	3	1	4	6
3	2	5	8	4	6	7	1	9
4	7	1	2	5	9	3	6	8
9	8	6	7	3	1	4	2	5
1	6	9	3	2	7	5	8	4
8	5	3	6	1	4	9	7	2
7	4	2	9	8	5	6	3	1

Sudoku Puzzle Solutions

Puzzle # 97

9	8	6	4	7	1	3	2	5
3	4	7	5	8	2	9	6	1
5	2	1	3	9	6	8	7	4
1	3	8	6	2	7	5	4	9
4	7	2	9	5	8	6	1	3
6	9	5	1	3	4	2	8	7
7	6	9	2	4	3	1	5	8
2	5	4	8	1	9	7	3	6
8	1	3	7	6	5	4	9	2

Puzzle # 98

7	5	6	4	1	9	3	2	8
9	8	1	3	2	7	5	6	4
3	4	2	5	8	6	9	1	7
5	2	7	9	4	1	6	8	3
6	1	3	2	7	8	4	9	5
8	9	4	6	3	5	1	7	2
1	3	5	8	9	2	7	4	6
2	6	9	7	5	4	8	3	1
4	7	8	1	6	3	2	5	9

Puzzle # 99

1	9	5	4	8	7	2	3	6
6	4	3	2	1	9	8	7	5
7	8	2	6	5	3	4	9	1
8	1	4	9	3	2	6	5	7
2	6	9	5	7	8	1	4	3
5	3	7	1	6	4	9	8	2
9	5	8	3	2	1	7	6	4
3	7	1	8	4	6	5	2	9
4	2	6	7	9	5	3	1	8

Puzzle # 100

3	6	7	1	8	9	2	4	5
2	5	9	4	7	6	3	1	8
1	4	8	2	5	3	7	6	9
9	8	6	7	3	2	1	5	4
5	7	3	8	4	1	6	9	2
4	1	2	9	6	5	8	7	3
8	9	4	6	2	7	5	3	1
7	2	5	3	1	4	9	8	6
6	3	1	5	9	8	4	2	7

Puzzle # 101

2	1	5	6	7	8	9	4	3
7	4	9	3	5	2	8	1	6
6	8	3	1	4	9	5	2	7
1	5	2	8	3	4	6	7	9
8	6	4	9	1	7	3	5	2
3	9	7	5	2	6	1	8	4
4	3	1	2	9	5	7	6	8
5	7	8	4	6	3	2	9	1
9	2	6	7	8	1	4	3	5

Puzzle # 102

4	9	6	2	1	3	5	8	7
7	2	8	6	4	5	1	9	3
1	3	5	8	9	7	4	2	6
8	1	7	5	3	9	2	6	4
2	6	4	1	7	8	3	5	9
9	5	3	4	2	6	8	7	1
3	7	2	9	5	1	6	4	8
6	4	1	7	8	2	9	3	5
5	8	9	3	6	4	7	1	2

Sudoku Puzzle Solutions

Puzzle # 103

6	1	9	5	7	3	8	2	4
3	4	2	6	8	1	5	7	9
7	8	5	4	2	9	1	3	6
9	5	7	2	4	8	6	1	3
8	6	3	9	1	7	4	5	2
4	2	1	3	5	6	7	9	8
2	7	6	8	3	5	9	4	1
5	9	4	1	6	2	3	8	7
1	3	8	7	9	4	2	6	5

Puzzle # 104

1	6	4	2	5	3	9	8	7
7	3	9	8	4	6	2	5	1
2	8	5	7	9	1	6	3	4
5	9	3	6	2	7	4	1	8
8	7	2	9	1	4	5	6	3
6	4	1	5	3	8	7	2	9
9	1	6	3	7	5	8	4	2
4	2	8	1	6	9	3	7	5
3	5	7	4	8	2	1	9	6

Puzzle # 105

7	2	4	1	3	8	5	6	9
5	9	8	2	7	6	3	4	1
6	1	3	5	4	9	2	8	7
4	5	7	6	8	2	9	1	3
1	6	2	9	5	3	8	7	4
8	3	9	7	1	4	6	2	5
2	8	1	3	9	7	4	5	6
3	4	5	8	6	1	7	9	2
9	7	6	4	2	5	1	3	8

Puzzle # 106

6	1	5	2	9	4	8	3	7
7	3	4	8	1	5	2	9	6
8	2	9	6	3	7	1	4	5
5	6	2	7	4	8	9	1	3
4	9	8	1	5	3	7	6	2
3	7	1	9	2	6	4	5	8
1	5	7	4	6	2	3	8	9
9	8	3	5	7	1	6	2	4
2	4	6	3	8	9	5	7	1

Puzzle # 107

4	5	6	8	3	9	1	7	2
3	9	7	5	1	2	4	6	8
2	1	8	6	7	4	3	9	5
7	4	9	1	8	3	5	2	6
5	8	2	4	9	6	7	1	3
6	3	1	2	5	7	9	8	4
8	2	3	9	4	1	6	5	7
9	6	4	7	2	5	8	3	1
1	7	5	3	6	8	2	4	9

Puzzle # 108

6	2	8	4	3	5	7	1	9
1	7	9	6	8	2	4	5	3
3	4	5	1	9	7	2	6	8
5	8	7	9	6	4	3	2	1
4	6	2	5	1	3	9	8	7
9	3	1	7	2	8	6	4	5
2	5	6	3	7	1	8	9	4
7	9	4	8	5	6	1	3	2
8	1	3	2	4	9	5	7	6

Sudoku Puzzle Solutions

Puzzle # 109

8	3	5	1	6	9	7	2	4
6	2	4	3	7	8	9	5	1
1	7	9	4	5	2	3	6	8
7	4	1	6	2	3	5	8	9
9	5	8	7	4	1	2	3	6
3	6	2	9	8	5	4	1	7
2	9	6	5	1	7	8	4	3
5	1	7	8	3	4	6	9	2
4	8	3	2	9	6	1	7	5

Puzzle # 110

6	8	3	7	5	4	1	9	2
7	5	9	6	2	1	4	3	8
1	2	4	3	8	9	7	6	5
5	9	1	2	4	3	6	8	7
4	7	2	8	1	6	9	5	3
3	6	8	9	7	5	2	1	4
8	3	7	1	9	2	5	4	6
9	4	6	5	3	7	8	2	1
2	1	5	4	6	8	3	7	9

Puzzle # 111

5	4	1	2	7	8	3	6	9
7	2	6	9	1	3	8	4	5
8	9	3	4	6	5	7	2	1
6	1	7	3	9	2	5	8	4
9	3	8	5	4	7	6	1	2
4	5	2	6	8	1	9	7	3
1	6	5	7	2	9	4	3	8
2	7	9	8	3	4	1	5	6
3	8	4	1	5	6	2	9	7

Puzzle # 112

9	5	4	7	2	1	3	8	6
8	7	6	3	5	4	2	9	1
2	3	1	8	6	9	7	4	5
6	2	5	1	4	8	9	7	3
4	8	3	9	7	5	6	1	2
1	9	7	6	3	2	8	5	4
7	1	2	5	9	6	4	3	8
5	6	9	4	8	3	1	2	7
3	4	8	2	1	7	5	6	9

Puzzle # 113

8	7	2	6	3	5	1	9	4
5	1	9	4	2	7	3	6	8
3	4	6	9	1	8	5	2	7
9	2	4	1	5	6	7	8	3
1	3	8	2	7	9	6	4	5
6	5	7	3	8	4	2	1	9
4	8	1	5	6	3	9	7	2
7	6	3	8	9	2	4	5	1
2	9	5	7	4	1	8	3	6

Puzzle # 114

1	8	6	3	5	2	4	7	9
9	7	2	8	1	4	3	6	5
4	5	3	6	7	9	8	1	2
8	4	5	9	6	3	1	2	7
6	3	1	7	2	8	5	9	4
2	9	7	1	4	5	6	8	3
5	6	9	4	8	7	2	3	1
7	2	8	5	3	1	9	4	6
3	1	4	2	9	6	7	5	8

Sudoku Puzzle Solutions

Puzzle # 115

9	1	7	8	2	5	3	4	6
3	4	8	7	9	6	2	5	1
2	6	5	4	3	1	8	9	7
5	2	4	1	8	3	6	7	9
6	3	9	2	5	7	1	8	4
7	8	1	9	6	4	5	3	2
1	5	6	3	4	9	7	2	8
8	9	3	6	7	2	4	1	5
4	7	2	5	1	8	9	6	3

Puzzle # 116

6	5	2	9	7	3	8	4	1
1	4	7	2	8	6	3	9	5
3	8	9	1	5	4	6	7	2
4	3	6	8	2	5	9	1	7
7	1	5	3	6	9	4	2	8
2	9	8	7	4	1	5	6	3
9	2	4	5	3	7	1	8	6
8	6	3	4	1	2	7	5	9
5	7	1	6	9	8	2	3	4

Puzzle # 117

2	4	7	5	3	1	9	6	8
6	1	9	8	4	7	5	2	3
8	3	5	9	6	2	7	1	4
5	6	3	7	8	9	2	4	1
9	2	1	4	5	6	3	8	7
7	8	4	1	2	3	6	9	5
3	9	8	6	1	5	4	7	2
4	7	2	3	9	8	1	5	6
1	5	6	2	7	4	8	3	9

Puzzle # 118

8	1	7	9	2	5	4	6	3
3	5	2	8	4	6	1	7	9
9	6	4	1	3	7	8	5	2
7	4	1	3	5	9	6	2	8
6	3	9	2	7	8	5	1	4
5	2	8	4	6	1	9	3	7
4	8	3	5	1	2	7	9	6
2	7	5	6	9	4	3	8	1
1	9	6	7	8	3	2	4	5

Puzzle # 119

1	7	2	8	4	5	9	3	6
5	9	6	1	2	3	7	8	4
3	8	4	9	6	7	1	5	2
4	2	5	7	1	9	3	6	8
9	6	8	4	3	2	5	7	1
7	3	1	5	8	6	4	2	9
8	1	7	2	5	4	6	9	3
6	4	9	3	7	8	2	1	5
2	5	3	6	9	1	8	4	7

Puzzle # 120

3	7	6	1	9	4	5	2	8
2	5	1	7	6	8	9	4	3
4	9	8	3	5	2	7	6	1
7	4	3	2	8	1	6	9	5
6	1	9	4	3	5	8	7	2
8	2	5	9	7	6	3	1	4
5	6	2	8	1	7	4	3	9
9	8	4	6	2	3	1	5	7
1	3	7	5	4	9	2	8	6

Sudoku Puzzle Solutions

Puzzle # 121

1	8	2	9	6	5	4	7	3
3	4	5	1	2	7	8	9	6
6	7	9	4	3	8	5	1	2
8	9	6	3	4	2	1	5	7
5	3	1	8	7	6	2	4	9
7	2	4	5	9	1	3	6	8
4	5	7	6	8	3	9	2	1
9	6	3	2	1	4	7	8	5
2	1	8	7	5	9	6	3	4

Puzzle # 122

6	9	8	7	2	5	3	4	1
2	7	4	6	1	3	8	9	5
5	1	3	8	4	9	6	7	2
7	2	9	4	3	1	5	8	6
8	4	6	2	5	7	1	3	9
1	3	5	9	6	8	7	2	4
9	8	1	5	7	4	2	6	3
4	5	2	3	8	6	9	1	7
3	6	7	1	9	2	4	5	8

Puzzle # 123

1	4	3	5	8	2	6	9	7
6	9	2	4	3	7	5	8	1
7	8	5	9	6	1	3	2	4
4	3	8	7	5	6	2	1	9
2	6	9	8	1	3	4	7	5
5	7	1	2	9	4	8	6	3
3	2	6	1	4	9	7	5	8
8	1	7	3	2	5	9	4	6
9	5	4	6	7	8	1	3	2

Puzzle # 124

6	9	2	4	1	5	3	7	8
4	8	3	9	2	7	5	6	1
1	5	7	8	6	3	4	9	2
2	4	1	7	8	6	9	3	5
5	3	6	1	9	2	7	8	4
9	7	8	5	3	4	2	1	6
7	6	9	2	4	1	8	5	3
8	1	4	3	5	9	6	2	7
3	2	5	6	7	8	1	4	9

Puzzle # 125

3	8	7	1	9	4	5	6	2
5	9	1	6	3	2	4	8	7
6	2	4	7	8	5	9	1	3
4	7	9	2	6	1	3	5	8
1	3	5	4	7	8	6	2	9
2	6	8	3	5	9	7	4	1
9	4	2	5	1	3	8	7	6
7	1	3	8	4	6	2	9	5
8	5	6	9	2	7	1	3	4

Puzzle # 126

1	9	5	6	4	3	8	7	2
2	6	4	7	8	9	5	1	3
3	8	7	5	1	2	9	4	6
6	5	9	3	7	8	1	2	4
8	3	1	9	2	4	7	6	5
7	4	2	1	5	6	3	9	8
5	7	6	2	3	1	4	8	9
4	2	3	8	9	7	6	5	1
9	1	8	4	6	5	2	3	7

Sudoku Puzzle Solutions

Puzzle # 127

2	5	6	8	3	1	9	7	4
1	3	9	4	6	7	5	8	2
8	7	4	5	9	2	3	1	6
4	6	1	3	2	8	7	5	9
5	8	3	9	7	6	4	2	1
9	2	7	1	4	5	8	6	3
3	1	8	6	5	4	2	9	7
7	9	5	2	1	3	6	4	8
6	4	2	7	8	9	1	3	5

Puzzle # 128

1	5	8	4	2	6	3	7	9
4	6	3	7	9	1	5	8	2
2	9	7	3	8	5	4	6	1
6	3	1	8	5	2	7	9	4
8	7	4	9	1	3	6	2	5
9	2	5	6	7	4	8	1	3
5	8	6	2	4	9	1	3	7
7	4	2	1	3	8	9	5	6
3	1	9	5	6	7	2	4	8

Puzzle # 129

4	7	5	8	3	2	6	9	1
2	8	3	6	9	1	4	5	7
9	1	6	7	5	4	8	3	2
7	4	9	3	6	5	2	1	8
6	3	1	9	2	8	7	4	5
8	5	2	1	4	7	9	6	3
1	9	4	2	7	3	5	8	6
5	2	8	4	1	6	3	7	9
3	6	7	5	8	9	1	2	4

Puzzle # 130

5	4	3	8	7	1	9	2	6
8	6	7	4	2	9	1	3	5
1	9	2	6	5	3	8	7	4
4	5	1	2	8	7	3	6	9
2	3	8	1	9	6	5	4	7
6	7	9	5	3	4	2	1	8
9	1	5	7	4	2	6	8	3
7	8	6	3	1	5	4	9	2
3	2	4	9	6	8	7	5	1

Puzzle # 131

8	2	1	5	6	4	3	9	7
6	4	7	9	3	8	1	5	2
5	3	9	2	1	7	4	6	8
3	1	2	7	5	6	9	8	4
9	6	5	8	4	1	2	7	3
4	7	8	3	9	2	6	1	5
7	9	4	1	8	3	5	2	6
2	5	3	6	7	9	8	4	1
1	8	6	4	2	5	7	3	9

Puzzle # 132

8	1	7	2	6	5	3	9	4
2	3	6	4	8	9	1	7	5
4	9	5	3	7	1	8	6	2
1	7	3	8	5	6	2	4	9
5	6	2	1	9	4	7	8	3
9	4	8	7	3	2	5	1	6
6	5	1	9	2	7	4	3	8
7	8	9	5	4	3	6	2	1
3	2	4	6	1	8	9	5	7

Sudoku Puzzle Solutions

Puzzle # 133

4	8	2	6	5	3	1	7	9
9	6	5	1	7	8	4	2	3
1	3	7	2	9	4	6	8	5
5	9	6	8	1	7	3	4	2
8	2	3	5	4	6	7	9	1
7	1	4	9	3	2	5	6	8
3	7	9	4	2	5	8	1	6
6	4	1	3	8	9	2	5	7
2	5	8	7	6	1	9	3	4

Puzzle # 134

2	8	3	7	1	5	6	9	4
9	7	1	6	8	4	2	5	3
6	5	4	9	2	3	7	8	1
5	3	7	1	6	9	4	2	8
1	2	9	4	3	8	5	6	7
8	4	6	5	7	2	3	1	9
3	6	5	8	9	7	1	4	2
4	9	2	3	5	1	8	7	6
7	1	8	2	4	6	9	3	5

Puzzle # 135

3	8	9	7	5	2	4	1	6
7	5	1	4	8	6	3	2	9
2	4	6	3	1	9	8	7	5
4	7	5	6	2	8	1	9	3
9	6	8	1	3	4	7	5	2
1	3	2	5	9	7	6	8	4
6	2	4	9	7	1	5	3	8
8	1	3	2	4	5	9	6	7
5	9	7	8	6	3	2	4	1

Puzzle # 136

6	7	3	5	1	2	8	4	9
4	8	2	6	9	3	5	1	7
5	1	9	7	8	4	3	6	2
7	6	4	3	2	9	1	8	5
9	2	8	1	5	6	7	3	4
3	5	1	4	7	8	2	9	6
1	3	5	9	4	7	6	2	8
8	9	7	2	6	1	4	5	3
2	4	6	8	3	5	9	7	1

Puzzle # 137

4	6	2	8	7	5	3	1	9
1	8	9	2	3	6	5	7	4
7	3	5	4	1	9	8	2	6
8	7	6	1	2	4	9	5	3
2	1	4	5	9	3	7	6	8
9	5	3	7	6	8	2	4	1
3	9	1	6	5	2	4	8	7
5	4	7	3	8	1	6	9	2
6	2	8	9	4	7	1	3	5

Puzzle # 138

7	2	6	5	8	4	9	1	3
3	8	9	1	2	7	5	4	6
4	5	1	9	6	3	8	2	7
9	3	8	7	5	1	2	6	4
5	4	2	3	9	6	1	7	8
1	6	7	8	4	2	3	9	5
2	7	3	4	1	5	6	8	9
6	9	4	2	3	8	7	5	1
8	1	5	6	7	9	4	3	2

Sudoku Puzzle Solutions

Puzzle # 139

3	9	1	2	8	5	4	6	7
7	4	8	9	1	6	2	3	5
5	6	2	7	3	4	1	9	8
1	8	6	5	2	7	9	4	3
9	7	4	3	6	1	5	8	2
2	3	5	4	9	8	6	7	1
6	2	9	1	7	3	8	5	4
4	1	7	8	5	9	3	2	6
8	5	3	6	4	2	7	1	9

Puzzle # 140

4	9	6	3	5	7	1	8	2
3	7	2	1	8	6	5	4	9
5	8	1	4	2	9	6	3	7
9	3	7	6	1	2	4	5	8
2	6	5	7	4	8	9	1	3
1	4	8	5	9	3	7	2	6
6	2	4	8	7	1	3	9	5
8	5	3	9	6	4	2	7	1
7	1	9	2	3	5	8	6	4

Puzzle # 141

5	2	1	9	4	3	7	6	8
8	7	6	5	2	1	3	4	9
3	4	9	6	8	7	1	5	2
2	6	7	3	5	9	8	1	4
4	1	3	2	7	8	5	9	6
9	5	8	1	6	4	2	3	7
7	9	4	8	3	5	6	2	1
1	3	2	7	9	6	4	8	5
6	8	5	4	1	2	9	7	3

Puzzle # 142

4	7	9	3	6	8	2	5	1
3	1	5	2	9	7	4	8	6
8	6	2	4	5	1	7	3	9
1	2	7	8	4	3	9	6	5
5	9	8	1	2	6	3	4	7
6	3	4	9	7	5	1	2	8
7	4	1	5	8	2	6	9	3
9	5	6	7	3	4	8	1	2
2	8	3	6	1	9	5	7	4

Puzzle # 143

7	9	3	4	1	5	2	6	8
6	1	2	7	8	9	5	3	4
4	8	5	6	3	2	7	9	1
1	6	4	2	7	3	9	8	5
3	2	7	9	5	8	4	1	6
8	5	9	1	4	6	3	2	7
9	3	1	5	6	4	8	7	2
5	7	8	3	2	1	6	4	9
2	4	6	8	9	7	1	5	3

Puzzle # 144

7	9	1	6	3	8	4	5	2
5	2	3	4	1	7	9	8	6
4	6	8	2	5	9	1	7	3
6	1	7	3	4	2	8	9	5
2	4	9	1	8	5	6	3	7
3	8	5	9	7	6	2	1	4
9	3	2	7	6	1	5	4	8
8	7	6	5	9	4	3	2	1
1	5	4	8	2	3	7	6	9

Sudoku Puzzle Solutions

Puzzle # 145

2	4	1	5	9	3	8	7	6
8	6	5	4	7	1	3	2	9
3	9	7	2	8	6	1	5	4
7	8	4	6	3	5	2	9	1
9	1	3	7	2	4	5	6	8
5	2	6	9	1	8	7	4	3
4	3	2	8	6	7	9	1	5
1	5	9	3	4	2	6	8	7
6	7	8	1	5	9	4	3	2

Puzzle # 146

6	8	4	1	7	3	5	2	9
7	1	2	5	9	6	4	8	3
5	9	3	4	2	8	1	7	6
8	3	6	9	4	7	2	1	5
2	5	9	8	6	1	3	4	7
4	7	1	2	3	5	9	6	8
3	4	5	7	8	2	6	9	1
9	6	7	3	1	4	8	5	2
1	2	8	6	5	9	7	3	4

Puzzle # 147

5	7	9	3	1	8	4	6	2
3	1	4	2	6	5	8	7	9
6	2	8	7	4	9	3	1	5
1	4	6	9	2	3	5	8	7
9	5	2	8	7	1	6	4	3
8	3	7	4	5	6	2	9	1
4	9	1	6	3	2	7	5	8
7	8	3	5	9	4	1	2	6
2	6	5	1	8	7	9	3	4

Puzzle # 148

3	7	6	1	8	5	9	2	4
5	9	1	4	3	2	6	8	7
2	4	8	7	9	6	1	5	3
9	6	2	5	7	3	8	4	1
8	1	5	6	2	4	7	3	9
4	3	7	9	1	8	2	6	5
1	8	4	3	6	7	5	9	2
6	5	9	2	4	1	3	7	8
7	2	3	8	5	9	4	1	6

Puzzle # 149

1	8	6	5	7	9	3	2	4
7	4	2	3	1	8	6	9	5
3	9	5	4	6	2	8	1	7
9	5	4	1	2	3	7	8	6
2	6	1	8	5	7	9	4	3
8	7	3	6	9	4	2	5	1
6	3	9	2	4	1	5	7	8
5	1	7	9	8	6	4	3	2
4	2	8	7	3	5	1	6	9

Puzzle # 150

3	8	6	5	1	7	9	4	2
4	5	2	3	8	9	7	1	6
9	7	1	2	4	6	3	8	5
5	3	8	9	2	1	6	7	4
1	9	4	7	6	5	2	3	8
6	2	7	4	3	8	1	5	9
8	6	5	1	9	3	4	2	7
7	4	3	6	5	2	8	9	1
2	1	9	8	7	4	5	6	3

Sudoku Puzzle Solutions

Puzzle # 151

2	9	5	8	1	4	3	7	6
7	6	1	5	3	9	4	8	2
8	3	4	7	2	6	5	1	9
3	2	9	4	7	8	1	6	5
4	5	8	9	6	1	7	2	3
6	1	7	2	5	3	9	4	8
5	4	2	3	8	7	6	9	1
9	8	6	1	4	5	2	3	7
1	7	3	6	9	2	8	5	4

Puzzle # 152

7	2	5	1	6	8	9	4	3
1	9	8	3	2	4	5	7	6
4	6	3	7	5	9	2	8	1
5	8	4	9	7	1	6	3	2
9	7	2	6	4	3	1	5	8
6	3	1	2	8	5	4	9	7
2	4	6	5	3	7	8	1	9
8	1	7	4	9	6	3	2	5
3	5	9	8	1	2	7	6	4

Puzzle # 153

7	9	4	6	5	1	8	3	2
2	1	3	9	4	8	6	5	7
8	6	5	2	7	3	9	4	1
5	7	6	1	8	2	3	9	4
1	3	2	5	9	4	7	8	6
4	8	9	7	3	6	2	1	5
9	4	7	8	2	5	1	6	3
6	5	8	3	1	7	4	2	9
3	2	1	4	6	9	5	7	8

Puzzle # 154

2	5	3	1	7	9	6	4	8
7	4	9	6	2	8	5	3	1
8	6	1	3	4	5	7	9	2
1	9	7	4	5	6	2	8	3
6	8	2	7	3	1	4	5	9
5	3	4	8	9	2	1	7	6
9	7	6	2	8	4	3	1	5
3	1	5	9	6	7	8	2	4
4	2	8	5	1	3	9	6	7

Puzzle # 155

6	5	8	9	3	1	4	7	2
1	2	7	8	5	4	3	6	9
3	4	9	7	2	6	5	1	8
2	6	1	5	4	8	7	9	3
7	8	5	3	6	9	2	4	1
9	3	4	2	1	7	6	8	5
5	9	6	1	7	2	8	3	4
8	7	3	4	9	5	1	2	6
4	1	2	6	8	3	9	5	7

Puzzle # 156

7	2	8	4	1	5	6	9	3
6	9	5	7	8	3	2	1	4
4	1	3	9	6	2	5	7	8
5	4	1	2	9	8	3	6	7
8	3	9	5	7	6	4	2	1
2	6	7	3	4	1	9	8	5
1	7	2	6	5	4	8	3	9
3	8	4	1	2	9	7	5	6
9	5	6	8	3	7	1	4	2

Sudoku Puzzle Solutions

Puzzle # 157

8	7	2	1	3	6	9	5	4
1	9	3	5	7	4	8	6	2
5	4	6	9	2	8	7	3	1
7	6	1	2	5	3	4	8	9
4	2	9	8	6	7	5	1	3
3	5	8	4	1	9	6	2	7
2	8	7	6	4	1	3	9	5
6	1	4	3	9	5	2	7	8
9	3	5	7	8	2	1	4	6

Puzzle # 158

3	8	7	6	2	4	9	5	1
6	9	1	7	5	8	4	3	2
2	5	4	9	3	1	6	7	8
5	2	3	8	1	9	7	4	6
4	7	9	2	6	5	8	1	3
8	1	6	3	4	7	2	9	5
7	4	5	1	8	6	3	2	9
1	3	8	4	9	2	5	6	7
9	6	2	5	7	3	1	8	4

Puzzle # 159

4	3	7	5	2	1	6	8	9
1	9	6	8	3	7	2	5	4
8	2	5	9	6	4	1	7	3
7	1	2	4	5	9	3	6	8
5	6	3	1	8	2	4	9	7
9	8	4	6	7	3	5	2	1
6	4	9	7	1	5	8	3	2
3	7	8	2	4	6	9	1	5
2	5	1	3	9	8	7	4	6

Puzzle # 160

2	3	6	7	8	9	5	4	1
9	1	5	2	3	4	7	6	8
8	4	7	5	6	1	9	3	2
4	6	1	3	5	7	8	2	9
5	2	8	9	1	6	4	7	3
7	9	3	8	4	2	6	1	5
3	7	9	6	2	8	1	5	4
6	5	4	1	9	3	2	8	7
1	8	2	4	7	5	3	9	6

Puzzle # 161

4	9	3	5	1	2	6	7	8
1	6	5	8	7	3	9	4	2
7	2	8	9	4	6	5	1	3
9	5	6	4	3	7	8	2	1
8	7	1	6	2	9	4	3	5
3	4	2	1	8	5	7	6	9
6	3	9	2	5	4	1	8	7
5	8	7	3	6	1	2	9	4
2	1	4	7	9	8	3	5	6

Puzzle # 162

5	1	2	3	6	7	9	8	4
6	7	8	2	9	4	1	5	3
4	9	3	8	5	1	2	6	7
3	8	1	4	7	9	6	2	5
2	5	4	6	1	3	8	7	9
7	6	9	5	8	2	3	4	1
1	3	5	7	2	8	4	9	6
8	4	6	9	3	5	7	1	2
9	2	7	1	4	6	5	3	8

Sudoku Puzzle Solutions

Puzzle # 163

6	2	9	5	1	7	4	3	8
8	3	7	9	4	2	5	1	6
1	5	4	6	3	8	7	2	9
7	9	1	8	5	4	3	6	2
2	6	3	1	7	9	8	4	5
4	8	5	2	6	3	1	9	7
3	7	8	4	9	6	2	5	1
9	1	2	3	8	5	6	7	4
5	4	6	7	2	1	9	8	3

Puzzle # 164

7	1	8	5	6	9	2	4	3
9	4	2	7	3	1	8	6	5
5	3	6	2	4	8	7	1	9
2	5	3	8	1	4	9	7	6
1	9	7	6	2	3	4	5	8
6	8	4	9	5	7	1	3	2
3	6	9	1	7	2	5	8	4
4	2	1	3	8	5	6	9	7
8	7	5	4	9	6	3	2	1

Puzzle # 165

5	8	7	2	1	6	3	9	4
3	4	6	7	8	9	5	2	1
9	1	2	3	5	4	8	7	6
4	5	8	9	6	1	2	3	7
2	7	1	4	3	8	9	6	5
6	3	9	5	2	7	1	4	8
1	9	5	6	4	3	7	8	2
8	6	3	1	7	2	4	5	9
7	2	4	8	9	5	6	1	3

Puzzle # 166

6	5	2	8	4	7	1	9	3
7	4	8	9	1	3	2	5	6
3	9	1	6	5	2	8	4	7
4	2	7	5	6	9	3	8	1
5	8	6	3	2	1	4	7	9
9	1	3	7	8	4	6	2	5
1	7	4	2	9	6	5	3	8
2	3	5	1	7	8	9	6	4
8	6	9	4	3	5	7	1	2

Puzzle # 167

6	9	7	4	3	5	2	8	1
3	4	1	2	8	6	7	9	5
8	2	5	7	1	9	3	4	6
2	6	4	5	9	8	1	7	3
5	7	3	1	4	2	8	6	9
1	8	9	3	6	7	4	5	2
4	5	2	6	7	1	9	3	8
9	3	6	8	2	4	5	1	7
7	1	8	9	5	3	6	2	4

Puzzle # 168

7	8	5	9	4	2	6	3	1
1	2	6	7	8	3	9	4	5
9	3	4	5	1	6	2	8	7
4	1	2	8	9	5	3	7	6
6	9	3	1	2	7	4	5	8
5	7	8	6	3	4	1	2	9
2	6	1	4	5	8	7	9	3
8	4	7	3	6	9	5	1	2
3	5	9	2	7	1	8	6	4

Sudoku Puzzle Solutions

Puzzle # 169

3	9	8	4	7	5	2	6	1
6	4	1	3	8	2	9	7	5
5	7	2	1	6	9	4	8	3
2	8	5	7	3	1	6	9	4
9	6	7	5	4	8	3	1	2
1	3	4	9	2	6	8	5	7
7	2	6	8	1	3	5	4	9
8	1	9	2	5	4	7	3	6
4	5	3	6	9	7	1	2	8

Puzzle # 170

9	4	8	1	7	6	5	3	2
1	2	5	9	3	4	8	7	6
6	7	3	5	8	2	4	1	9
2	8	1	3	5	7	9	6	4
4	9	7	6	2	1	3	8	5
3	5	6	4	9	8	7	2	1
7	3	4	2	6	9	1	5	8
5	1	2	8	4	3	6	9	7
8	6	9	7	1	5	2	4	3

Puzzle # 171

4	6	1	8	7	5	9	2	3
5	8	7	3	9	2	4	1	6
9	3	2	6	1	4	7	5	8
7	2	5	9	8	6	3	4	1
3	9	4	5	2	1	6	8	7
6	1	8	4	3	7	5	9	2
1	4	9	7	6	8	2	3	5
8	7	3	2	5	9	1	6	4
2	5	6	1	4	3	8	7	9

Puzzle # 172

6	4	1	5	2	8	7	3	9
8	3	2	9	7	6	1	4	5
5	7	9	3	1	4	8	6	2
1	9	3	2	4	5	6	8	7
2	8	7	6	9	1	4	5	3
4	5	6	7	8	3	2	9	1
7	1	4	8	3	9	5	2	6
9	2	5	4	6	7	3	1	8
3	6	8	1	5	2	9	7	4

Puzzle # 173

7	9	1	3	6	4	2	5	8
8	5	2	7	9	1	6	4	3
4	6	3	5	8	2	9	7	1
1	7	6	2	5	9	8	3	4
9	2	4	8	3	7	1	6	5
5	3	8	1	4	6	7	9	2
3	1	9	6	2	5	4	8	7
6	8	7	4	1	3	5	2	9
2	4	5	9	7	8	3	1	6

Puzzle # 174

2	6	9	7	4	3	5	8	1
1	8	5	2	9	6	7	4	3
3	7	4	5	1	8	9	6	2
6	4	7	3	2	1	8	9	5
5	3	1	4	8	9	6	2	7
8	9	2	6	7	5	1	3	4
9	2	3	8	5	7	4	1	6
7	1	6	9	3	4	2	5	8
4	5	8	1	6	2	3	7	9

Sudoku Puzzle Solutions

Puzzle # 175

8	7	5	1	9	4	2	3	6
6	2	4	3	7	5	8	9	1
3	9	1	8	2	6	4	7	5
2	5	3	4	6	7	9	1	8
7	1	9	2	8	3	5	6	4
4	6	8	9	5	1	7	2	3
9	3	2	5	1	8	6	4	7
5	4	7	6	3	2	1	8	9
1	8	6	7	4	9	3	5	2

Puzzle # 176

8	1	3	6	5	2	4	7	9
4	5	2	3	7	9	1	8	6
9	7	6	1	8	4	2	5	3
3	4	9	5	6	7	8	1	2
5	6	7	8	2	1	3	9	4
1	2	8	4	9	3	5	6	7
7	8	4	9	3	5	6	2	1
6	9	1	2	4	8	7	3	5
2	3	5	7	1	6	9	4	8

Puzzle # 177

1	9	3	4	6	2	5	7	8
5	7	8	9	1	3	4	6	2
4	2	6	7	8	5	3	1	9
7	3	1	2	9	4	6	8	5
2	6	5	1	7	8	9	3	4
9	8	4	5	3	6	7	2	1
3	1	2	6	4	9	8	5	7
6	5	9	8	2	7	1	4	3
8	4	7	3	5	1	2	9	6

Puzzle # 178

8	2	1	9	7	4	5	6	3
4	3	5	2	6	1	9	8	7
9	7	6	3	5	8	2	1	4
7	8	2	5	3	6	4	9	1
5	1	3	4	8	9	7	2	6
6	4	9	7	1	2	8	3	5
3	6	4	8	2	5	1	7	9
1	9	8	6	4	7	3	5	2
2	5	7	1	9	3	6	4	8

Puzzle # 179

8	1	2	5	3	9	7	4	6
9	7	6	1	2	4	3	5	8
5	3	4	7	6	8	2	9	1
1	4	5	3	8	7	9	6	2
7	2	3	6	9	5	1	8	4
6	8	9	2	4	1	5	3	7
3	6	1	4	5	2	8	7	9
2	5	8	9	7	6	4	1	3
4	9	7	8	1	3	6	2	5

Puzzle # 180

6	3	9	8	1	2	5	7	4
1	2	7	4	5	6	9	3	8
4	5	8	7	3	9	1	6	2
5	6	3	1	4	7	2	8	9
8	9	2	5	6	3	4	1	7
7	4	1	2	9	8	3	5	6
3	7	6	9	2	1	8	4	5
2	8	5	3	7	4	6	9	1
9	1	4	6	8	5	7	2	3

Sudoku Puzzle Solutions

Puzzle # 181

6	5	9	7	2	4	3	1	8
8	2	3	5	6	1	7	4	9
7	1	4	8	3	9	2	5	6
1	6	8	3	5	7	9	2	4
2	9	7	4	8	6	5	3	1
4	3	5	9	1	2	6	8	7
3	8	1	6	7	5	4	9	2
5	4	6	2	9	8	1	7	3
9	7	2	1	4	3	8	6	5

Puzzle # 182

5	4	2	7	9	3	6	8	1
7	8	6	1	5	4	9	2	3
3	1	9	6	8	2	4	5	7
6	5	4	3	2	9	7	1	8
9	2	1	8	7	6	3	4	5
8	3	7	5	4	1	2	9	6
2	6	3	9	1	5	8	7	4
1	9	8	4	3	7	5	6	2
4	7	5	2	6	8	1	3	9

Puzzle # 183

2	1	8	3	9	6	5	4	7
4	5	3	8	1	7	6	2	9
7	9	6	5	4	2	3	8	1
5	6	2	1	8	4	9	7	3
8	7	4	6	3	9	2	1	5
1	3	9	2	7	5	4	6	8
3	2	7	9	6	1	8	5	4
6	8	1	4	5	3	7	9	2
9	4	5	7	2	8	1	3	6

Puzzle # 184

9	3	1	8	4	5	7	2	6
5	2	7	9	3	6	8	1	4
8	6	4	1	2	7	9	3	5
2	7	3	6	1	8	4	5	9
1	8	9	2	5	4	6	7	3
4	5	6	7	9	3	1	8	2
6	1	5	4	8	2	3	9	7
7	9	2	3	6	1	5	4	8
3	4	8	5	7	9	2	6	1

Puzzle # 185

9	3	8	1	2	5	6	4	7
1	4	6	8	7	9	5	2	3
7	2	5	3	6	4	9	1	8
6	9	4	2	8	7	3	5	1
8	7	1	6	5	3	4	9	2
2	5	3	9	4	1	7	8	6
4	8	7	5	3	2	1	6	9
5	1	2	7	9	6	8	3	4
3	6	9	4	1	8	2	7	5

Puzzle # 186

6	5	9	4	3	8	1	2	7
1	4	8	7	5	2	3	9	6
7	3	2	9	6	1	4	5	8
2	9	6	1	7	3	5	8	4
3	1	5	6	8	4	9	7	2
4	8	7	5	2	9	6	1	3
8	6	3	2	9	5	7	4	1
9	2	4	3	1	7	8	6	5
5	7	1	8	4	6	2	3	9

Sudoku Puzzle Solutions

Puzzle # 187

8	4	9	7	5	3	2	6	1
1	3	5	2	8	6	9	7	4
7	2	6	4	9	1	5	3	8
6	9	2	1	3	8	7	4	5
4	7	8	5	6	2	1	9	3
3	5	1	9	4	7	6	8	2
5	1	3	6	7	4	8	2	9
2	8	7	3	1	9	4	5	6
9	6	4	8	2	5	3	1	7

Puzzle # 188

9	8	4	1	2	5	3	7	6
2	6	7	4	9	3	1	8	5
1	3	5	7	8	6	4	2	9
4	9	6	8	3	1	2	5	7
3	7	8	5	6	2	9	4	1
5	1	2	9	4	7	8	6	3
7	4	9	6	1	8	5	3	2
6	2	1	3	5	4	7	9	8
8	5	3	2	7	9	6	1	4

Puzzle # 189

5	7	4	6	1	8	9	3	2
2	8	1	9	3	7	5	4	6
6	3	9	4	5	2	1	7	8
1	9	3	8	6	4	7	2	5
4	6	2	5	7	3	8	9	1
8	5	7	1	2	9	3	6	4
9	2	6	7	8	5	4	1	3
7	1	5	3	4	6	2	8	9
3	4	8	2	9	1	6	5	7

Puzzle # 190

3	1	2	7	6	4	5	9	8
6	4	7	5	8	9	3	1	2
5	8	9	1	2	3	6	4	7
9	7	4	2	5	6	1	8	3
2	5	8	9	3	1	7	6	4
1	6	3	4	7	8	2	5	9
8	9	5	3	1	7	4	2	6
4	3	1	6	9	2	8	7	5
7	2	6	8	4	5	9	3	1

Puzzle # 191

5	6	1	8	3	7	4	9	2
9	7	8	4	2	5	1	6	3
3	2	4	9	6	1	8	5	7
1	5	3	7	4	8	6	2	9
7	4	2	6	5	9	3	1	8
6	8	9	2	1	3	5	7	4
8	1	7	3	9	6	2	4	5
4	9	5	1	8	2	7	3	6
2	3	6	5	7	4	9	8	1

Puzzle # 192

1	6	3	8	9	2	7	4	5
5	4	8	3	1	7	9	2	6
7	2	9	4	5	6	1	8	3
3	1	5	2	8	4	6	7	9
4	7	2	5	6	9	8	3	1
8	9	6	1	7	3	2	5	4
6	8	4	9	2	5	3	1	7
2	3	7	6	4	1	5	9	8
9	5	1	7	3	8	4	6	2

Sudoku Puzzle Solutions

Puzzle # 193

2	4	7	8	9	3	5	1	6
6	5	1	7	2	4	3	8	9
9	8	3	1	6	5	7	2	4
5	9	8	2	3	1	4	6	7
1	2	4	5	7	6	9	3	8
7	3	6	9	4	8	2	5	1
3	7	9	6	8	2	1	4	5
4	6	5	3	1	7	8	9	2
8	1	2	4	5	9	6	7	3

Puzzle # 194

1	5	3	7	8	4	2	6	9
4	2	9	3	1	6	5	7	8
7	8	6	2	9	5	3	4	1
5	4	2	9	6	1	8	3	7
6	9	7	8	3	2	4	1	5
3	1	8	4	5	7	6	9	2
2	7	1	6	4	8	9	5	3
9	6	5	1	2	3	7	8	4
8	3	4	5	7	9	1	2	6

Puzzle # 195

7	3	1	9	2	4	6	5	8
6	5	4	1	7	8	9	2	3
9	8	2	3	5	6	1	7	4
4	7	6	5	1	2	3	8	9
5	9	8	7	6	3	4	1	2
1	2	3	8	4	9	7	6	5
3	4	7	2	8	1	5	9	6
8	6	5	4	9	7	2	3	1
2	1	9	6	3	5	8	4	7

Puzzle # 196

5	7	3	1	9	6	4	8	2
2	4	6	8	7	3	1	9	5
1	9	8	2	4	5	7	6	3
6	5	7	3	1	9	2	4	8
9	2	4	7	5	8	6	3	1
8	3	1	6	2	4	5	7	9
3	1	5	4	8	7	9	2	6
7	8	2	9	6	1	3	5	4
4	6	9	5	3	2	8	1	7

Puzzle # 197

1	3	6	2	4	7	5	8	9
7	4	5	3	9	8	2	6	1
9	8	2	1	5	6	7	3	4
4	5	1	7	2	3	6	9	8
2	6	3	9	8	5	1	4	7
8	9	7	4	6	1	3	5	2
5	7	9	8	3	2	4	1	6
6	2	4	5	1	9	8	7	3
3	1	8	6	7	4	9	2	5

Puzzle # 198

8	2	4	1	6	3	7	5	9
6	5	9	8	7	2	1	4	3
3	1	7	9	4	5	2	8	6
1	6	8	3	2	4	9	7	5
9	7	3	5	8	1	6	2	4
5	4	2	6	9	7	8	3	1
4	9	6	7	3	8	5	1	2
2	8	5	4	1	6	3	9	7
7	3	1	2	5	9	4	6	8

Sudoku Puzzle Solutions

Puzzle # 199

4	7	5	1	8	2	3	9	6
2	8	6	9	3	4	7	1	5
3	1	9	7	6	5	8	2	4
8	9	3	6	4	1	2	5	7
1	5	2	8	9	7	4	6	3
6	4	7	2	5	3	1	8	9
7	3	1	5	2	6	9	4	8
9	6	4	3	1	8	5	7	2
5	2	8	4	7	9	6	3	1

Puzzle # 200

3	4	9	7	6	8	5	1	2
2	5	7	3	4	1	6	9	8
8	1	6	5	9	2	7	3	4
5	6	3	1	2	4	9	8	7
9	7	8	6	5	3	4	2	1
1	2	4	8	7	9	3	5	6
6	9	2	4	1	5	8	7	3
7	8	1	9	3	6	2	4	5
4	3	5	2	8	7	1	6	9

www.ingramcontent.com/pod-product-compliance
Lightning Source LLC
Chambersburg PA
CBHW052035280526
45791CB00010B/2972